when you want to say yes,
but your body says no

when you want to say yes, but your body says no

The Proven Mind-Body Plan to Beat Chronic Fatigue and Stress-related Illness

LIZ TUCKER

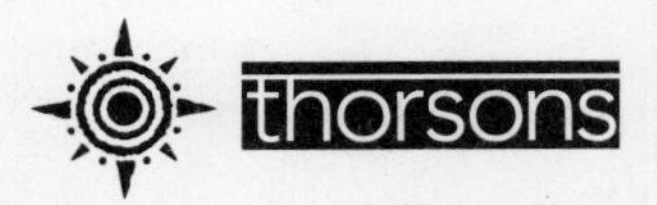

Thorsons
An Imprint of HarperCollins*Publishers*
77–85 Fulham Palace Road
Hammersmith, London W6 8JB

The website address is: www.thorsonselement.com

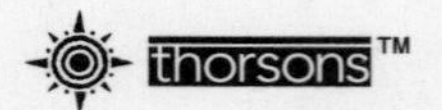

and *Thorsons* are trademarks of
HarperCollins*Publishers* Ltd

First published by Thorsons 2003

3 5 7 9 10 8 6 4

A catalogue record of this book is
available from the British Library

ISBN 0 00 715510 7

Printed and bound in Great Britain by
Creative Print and Design (Wales), Ebbw Vale

contents

foreword

Dr Sarah Brewer

I have heard Liz speak at health shows on a number of occasions and am always impressed by how she relates to her audience, taking them straight to the root of the problem and giving a number of well-thought out solutions. Her quick fixes are particularly useful.

Liz has discovered that most of the people she helps have two common failings – a lack of understanding about how they have arrived at the situation they are in, and a lack of preparation in their attempts to resolve their problem. As she points out, for your body to say *yes*, you must first find out why it is saying *no*. Liz helps you to become your own health detective, so you can find out what is wrong and take steps to get back on the right path. She shows you how to work through the sources of stress in your life, recognize the physical and emotional warning signs of overload, and change the way you think, turning things around so you can have a more positive outlook on life. This is an excellent introduction to self help and is bound to become a well-thumbed 'bible' for many people.

introduction

What's Your Problem?

Why is it that we are capable of dreaming up ambitious wants and desires that seem achievable yet, as soon as we put our mind and body in gear, mental fears and physical obstacles appear that prevent us going any further?

You would expect the body and mind to want what is best for us, so why do they seem to conspire against us when all we want to do is improve on a situation that is making us unhappy or unhealthy? We find it impossible to lose weight because although we want to eat healthily and get fit, our mind says let's eat more chocolate and our body refuses to enjoy exercise. We would like to do more with our life but our mind tells us to keep watching the television and our body agrees. We would like to have a less stressful daily schedule but our mind tells us we must keep going while our body runs out of energy and wants to stop.

So why does this happen? The answer is surprisingly simple. It happens because we are thinking solely about our own requirements and not considering that our body has a list of demands all of its own. If you are proposing to do something and you need some bodily assistance, then you have to convince your body that what you want to do will not be detrimental to its long-term health and well-being. In addition, your body has to feel confident that it has enough resources and the ability to see the task through. If your body feels under-resourced and concerned that the effort could be detrimental, it is not going to encourage you to continue and will sabotage any efforts you make.

When I was ill with ME, all I wanted to do was to get back to the lifestyle I had before I became ill. Despite the fact that my body had virtually lost its ability to function, I refused to see this as my body's way of telling me that it certainly didn't like that lifestyle. My turning point came when I eventually acknowledged that I needed to completely redesign my method for living if I wanted to live any sort of life at all. This change in attitude completely altered my prospects of recovery because I started working with my body and not against it.

My problem was an all too common one – I assumed that I could do what I wanted and my body would put up with it. Its function is, after all, to meet my demands. My downfall was a result of pure ignorance. I knew absolutely nothing about how my body worked and what it required to function effectively. I had no idea that the body has a very specific way it likes to be run and that the negative symptoms that I was experiencing, such as pain and fatigue, were warning signs that this was not happening. I demanded and expected the maximum out of my body without even considering that it needed time to rest and repair. I also never gave a moment's thought to the fact that nutrition and fluid are, without sounding too dramatic, the things that keep us alive – I ate junk food because I liked it and never drank water because it was boring.

Be Your Own Health Detective

Finding my route to recovery was a result of some thorough detective work – I looked at my symptoms, lifestyle and attitude in a search for clues to my ill health. It is this same process that you need to go through to uncover your own recovery route. If your body is not doing what you what it to do, then you need to look at what is making it so resistant to your demands. If you want to improve your health and happiness, you need to become your own health detective. By following the clues and sifting through the evidence you will have every chance of discovering what is at the root of your problems.

My first step forward came when I recognized that I was an individual and that this meant that general health advice didn't always work for *me*. If blanket health rules worked for all of us then we would all be happy and healthy as a result of getting the recommended amount of exercise, fruit and vegetables and water per day. Although the advice is generally beneficial, this does not mean it will work for everyone. It is aimed at the majority and by its very nature cannot consider individual requirements. For example, foods such as fruit, cereals and dairy produce are recommended as part of a healthy diet but, for a minority, they can create health problems. Similarly, you need to question why – if you are aware of ways of improving your health through diet, exercise or stress reduction – you choose not to follow this advice.

There is only one sure indicator that any advice is beneficial to you and that is that you receive positive results from implementing it. However, there is so much health advice available today, where do you start?

This book is designed to show you how, like me, you can uncover your own route to better health and happiness. Its purpose is not to dictate what will and won't work, but to help you find what will and won't work for you as an individual. You are the only one that can make a difference to your health and happiness because you are the only one that knows what will really work for you, based on the results you achieve. Only by taking control of your own health and well-being can you have any hope of changing the things you want to change and living the life that you want to live.

Getting The Best Out Of This Book

This book is designed to help you through the process of 'health detection', with tips, information and plans that will make it easier for you take to control of your own health and well-being. The aim is to encourage you to try things out so that you can see what works best for you. It should be read in sequence and, because it is not a passive experience, there are exercises for you to do and questions for you to answer. One of the things that really helped me to good health was gaining a greater understanding of how the body works. This enabled me to locate the cause of mysterious symptoms, detect the connection between seemingly unrelated problems and to analyse more successfully the variety of advice I was given. You need that same background knowledge, so you will find lots of information on how the body works.

If you feel that life would be better if you just had more energy or could control chronic health conditions, then part one is particularly appropriate to you as it looks closely at the physical aspects of poor health. If you feel stuck in a rut of repeated setbacks or your problems stem more from an emotional angle, then part two will prove invaluable. However, do remember the holistic approach – very few of us have a physical or mental issue without it affecting the rest of the body and mind to some extent. That is why this book looks into total physical health and mental well-being – because without one it's hard to maintain the other.

A Healthier Understanding

Part one, Body Intelligence, discusses how the body works and how it likes to be run. It provides knowledge that, albeit basic, can make a big difference to how you deal with your health. It looks at how a healthy body operates and how easy it is to upset the system. If we follow the route to ill health we can then retrace our steps back to a healthier existence. By listening more to your body and understanding what the negative signs mean, you can make better choices about your health and well-being.

Part one concentrates on the physical demands of the body but it also demonstrates how these can affect your mental well-being. It is impossible to separate physical and mental health issues. We all know that if we have a physical injury, a negative mental response will follow. Similarly, if we are unhappy, then we will notice an increase in physical symptoms such as fatigue and pain. It is all about balance. The body has a healthy balance that it likes to maintain but this requires constant monitoring and maintenance. Part one will help you find your healthy balance, and an incentive for doing so. When the body is unhappy it will tell you via negative mental responses and physical symptoms but when it is happy it will reward you with lots of positive feedback to encourage you to keep things that way.

Symptoms Of 'Unwellness'

If you have health problems, it is vital that your first port of call is your doctor. Doctors have a vast pool of knowledge and resources available for the purpose of improving *your* health, so don't be reluctant to use them. And don't feel that you need to feel really ill before you can justify a visit – feeling 'unwell' rather than 'ill' is an indication that your health is going downhill and a visit to your doctor may just help prevent a further deterioration. If you have symptoms that prove to be un-diagnosable and chronic, the chances are they will be more to do with lifestyle than a disease or illness – but that doesn't mean that they won't eventually turn into an illness if they are not addressed at an early stage.

The usual path to ill health goes something like this:

HEALTHY to UNHEALTHY to UNWELL to ILL to CHRONIC CONDITION to DIAGNOSABLE ILLNESS to CHRONIC ILLNESS

The problem with a diagnosable illness is that its effects may be irreversible so you may well be faced with the prospect of management rather than cure. However, chronic conditions can be managed very successfully. I myself suffer from one and, with good management, I experience hardly any problems at all. In fact, it only rears its ugly head when I get too run down or if I ease up on my maintenance – a flare-up is always a good indicator that I'm letting things slip and a great motivator to put things right.

In contrast, feeling unhealthy may not be something a doctor can diagnose but it is something that you can address – so start looking at how you can help yourself. Look at the symptoms outlined below and write down any that relate to you and any others that you suffer from.

Common Symptoms

Fatigue

- Do you suffer from fatigue that is chronic, constant, fluctuating, unexplainable or that occurs at set times during the day?
- Do you have trouble sleeping, even when you are tired, or do you feel you could sleep all the time?

Skeletal

- Do you get aches in your joints when you move and, when you don't move, burning sensations or discomfort?

Muscular

- Do your muscles hurt when touched, have no power, feel restless or give out sharp pains when you move?

Nerves

- Are you over-emotional or do you feel completely disinterested, even in those you love?

- Do you have a low pain threshold or do you get numbness or pins and needles in your hands and feet?

Cranial
- Are you very forgetful, accident-prone, find it hard to concentrate or have a short attention span?

Senses
- Do you get blurred vision, misunderstand what people say, have a poor sense of smell or only taste the flavour of very spicy foods.

Hormonal
- Do you get over-anxious, suffer from lethargy, find it hard to maintain a steady weight or experience mood changes that relate to your environment?

Skin
- Do you suffer from dry, flaky or inflamed skin, unexplained rashes or inflammation or is your skin sensitive to certain substances or to touch?

Cardiovascular
- Do you suffer from high blood pressure, palpitations, flushing skin, dizziness or poor circulation?

Immune system
- Do you seem to get every virus going, have you always got a cold, find it hard to recover from an illness or find that injuries are slow to heal?

Lungs
- Do you suffer from shortness of breath, wheezing, irritating coughs or low excursion levels?

Digestive
- Do you suffer from bloating, abdominal pains, food cravings, weight problems or acid reflux?

Urinary
- Do you get pains in the middle of your back, bladder discomfort, incontinence or regular bouts of cystitis?

Gynaecological
- Do you suffer from problem periods, thrush, painful sex or reproductive disorders?

All these symptoms can be generated by your lifestyle, environment, diet or some small physical imbalance that may be impossible to detect at an early stage with medical methods of diagnosis – although that doesn't mean that it is untreatable. With the exception of fatigue (which is the most universal symptom of being unhealthy and the most likely to appear first), I have grouped symptoms into the systems of the body they are likely to manifest in. However, this does not mean that they are not interlinked with, or even generated from, other systems in the body. This is why it is so important to address the overall health of the body and not treat symptoms in isolation. Having written down all those symptoms that relate to you, and any others you may suffer from, you now have your first set of clues. Part one of this book will help you unravel some of the mystery of the body with the aim of enabling you to relate this back to your particular health problems.

Making A Start

Part two, Changing Your Mind, is all about preparing to change. One of the biggest causes of anxiety is being aware that something is wrong but not knowing how to change it. When this occurs, you feel miserable because you feel trapped in a negative environment and frustrated that you cannot see a way out. As time passes, the gap between where you are and where you want to be often appears to grow wider. Part two looks at why, if you are so unhappy in a situation, you choose to remain in it.

Careful preparation will increase your chances of success dramatically and will reduce the fear factor. It will also provide you with a safe environment to experiment and recognize your true incentives. We only change if we have a very good incentive to do so and many plans fail because this is not acknowledged from the outset.

I did say that this is not a passive experience. This book offers support and will act as a fact finder, motivator and organizer. However, it will not change your life – *you* need to do that bit and it will involve effort. If you cringed at that last word, try to see effort in a more positive light – it doesn't need to be unpleasant. Effort should be stimulating and satisfying; an experience that ends on a high when you reach your goal. Unfortunately we often put a lot of pointless effort into things that bring little reward. It is not surprising then, that we perceive any effort as dull and mundane. If you want success, you need to forget about what you already think and do, because your existing approach isn't working.

If you feel stuck in a rut, this will be reflected in your attitude and thought patterns. Part two encourages you to look outside your normal conceptions and offers new ways of addressing problems.

10 Questions To Ask Yourself

Do you feel guilty about being unhappy with your life?
Do you find it hard to motivate yourself?
Do you feel tired all the time?
Do you lack confidence and self-esteem?

Have you had repeated problems for a prolonged period of time?
When was the last time you really laughed out loud?
Are the people around you a constant source of disappointment?
Do you think that life could be so much better if you could only resolve one negative issue?
Do you suffer from constant anxiety and stress?
Do you think it is possible to improve your situation?

If any of these questions strike a chord with how you are feeling now then get a pen and paper and write down all the reasons why you feel this way and how these things affect your life. It is important that you give honest answers because these will be your starting point for changing your situation, your benchmark for what you want to achieve. Part two will help you re-examine your existing approach and point you in the direction of some better answers.

Putting It All Together

Once you have done the preparation in parts one and two, all you need to do is put all your new-found knowledge into practice. Part three, Plan For Success, is all about making things happen. If you want success, you need to build in time to make it happen and the way to do this is to follow a custom-built strategy. In many aspects of our practical lives, like work or childcare for example, we are successful because we have to follow deadlines, assess priorities and produce results. We often have a problem achieving more fundamental requirements – for example, experiencing pleasure, love, good health and satisfaction – because we do not apply the same successful planning. If you do not set aside time for pleasure, for maintaining your body and concentrating on what really is important to you, if you disregard your need for personal satisfaction and success, then it really should be no surprise that you are unhappy. The same goes for your physical health. We often say that health is the most important thing in our life but, in reality, a great many of us give it little priority.

Life is a mix of mundane chores, difficult situations and pleasurable moments. By planning, you have a better chance of isolating and dealing with the mundane, reducing and coping with the difficult, and increasing and benefiting from the pleasurable – and keeping yourself in the best health possible.

To begin the process of change, you need to assess the situation you are in now. The questions and exercises in parts one and two are designed to help you examine your current situation. Practical guidance and information are provided to enable you to discover new ways of approaching and dealing with your own individual problems. Part three shows you how to put together all that you have discovered about yourself and helps you formulate that information into a usable plan that will enable you to make progress in combating your problem. By looking at your current reality, you can objectively separate the good from the bad. This book will help you sift through the clutter of your life as it is now, with the aim of clearing a path to an improved life. Learning to prioritize, prepare, detect, experiment, assess and acknowledge existing positive components in your life will help you focus on building a better future.

Part One

body intelligence

In order to get your body to say yes, you must first find out why it is saying no. Your body is your machine for living and if there are problems with the running of that machine, negative symptoms such as pain and fatigue will be generated. However, because the simple act of living results in wear and tear, both emotional and physical, the human body has an in-built repair and maintenance system. This system is so effective that it is capable of dealing with an extraordinary amount of abuse – but only if it is in good working order.

Health problems occur when this system develops a fault or fails due to:

- overload
- lengthy exposure to an ongoing problem
- damage
- a natural flaw or weakness

Overload

This often occurs when a combination of emotional and physical pressures are experienced at the same time, such as redundancy, relationship breakdown, an illness or injury and moving house. The body could probably cope with these issues individually but experiencing a catalogue of trauma all in one go can prove to be more than it can bear.

Ongoing Problems

An ongoing physical or emotional stress or anxiety that has been occurring for a long period of time – for instance, years of poor posture, deprivation of essential nutrients from a restrictive or poor diet or being disliked by your mother-in-law during 10 years of marriage – can lead to illness. Even if the stress is small, the constant drip, drip, drip of anxiety puts an additional strain on the body's ability to deal with the stresses of day-to-day living.

Damage

Any illness, injury or emotional trauma, such as an accident or a bereavement, can have a wide-ranging effect. Recent research has shown that almost one in two people do not fully recover from a minor illness or injury. This means that each one we experience leaves our body weaker and less able to cope with the next.

Flaws Or Weaknesses

These can result from a genetic or inherent health problem or from lack of use – for instance, poor muscle tone due to lack of movement or a weak bladder caused by years of dehydration. If you suffer from a flaw or weakness, you need to take extra special care of your body and work on improving your capabilities rather than fighting against your restriction.

Many of the causes of ill health outlined above are regarded as 'lifestyle' problems. However, they do have physical effects and these can be difficult to medically diagnose. For this reason, such illnesses are often labelled as psychological – despite the fact that the patient feels very real physical symptoms and is often only depressed as a direct result of their symptoms.

When I was ill, there was no doubt in my mind that my health problems were physical. My life before my burnout was exciting and I liked to live it to the maximum. I thrived on problem solving and achievement, and always focused on the positive and constructive rather than dwelling on the negative. I did suffer from chronic health problems but was determined not to let them affect my life – I thought there was no need to, as I appeared to have endless amounts of energy. Like so many, I had aspired to this lifestyle because I wanted a life that was stimulating and satisfying.

When I became really ill, it seemed obvious to me that the cause had to be physical because when I had first become ill my mental state could not have been brighter. I was amazed when no one could explain why I was so ill, diagnose me with something and treat it. I was also bewildered as to why I was being bombarded with questions about my mental state. Of course I had anxieties and depressing thoughts – who wouldn't if they were incapable of doing any of the things they loved? – but this did not mean I had suffered from them in the past. Okay, so there had been a huge amount of stress and activity in my life but very few of the causal factors were negative. In fact, the only negative thing in my life at the time was my on-going physical health condition.

If the experts could find no physical reason for my illness then I was happy to go along with their prognosis of a mental breakdown – I just wanted to get better and resume my past life because this one was no fun at all. When anti-depressants made me depressed and psychiatrists concluded that my mind was 'very positive under the circumstances', I was filed under the ME, chronic fatigue, post viral, burnout, breakdown category and told to just wait and see. No one dare mention that my lifestyle had anything to do with my illness. My medical experts were very good and very thorough but they could not help me because my problems could not be found in their system of diagnosis. Medical professionals are health detectives. They are no different to you or me, just much better informed. They wanted to help me but just didn't know how. It was obvious that I was ill but technically I was not because their system of diagnosis couldn't come up with anything.

If their detection process was not showing results then I would have to look for new clues myself. What I very quickly discovered was the extent of my ignorance – I didn't know the first thing about keeping my body healthy. I had always suffered from chronic health problems and now I had no energy either. I knew so little about keeping my body alive that I had been unwittingly killing it off. I was so ill that if a doctor had told me that most of my problems were down to my own ignorance and excesses and that it was nothing more than too much of everything for too long, I would have been furious – so it's no surprise that none of them ever did.

When I learnt for myself how the body works and likes to be run it became obvious why I had been so ill and, therefore, how I could put it right. This is what I want to help you achieve – a greater understanding of how to keep your body happy and healthy. I can see now that my body has natural weaknesses that generated my health problems. However, instead of giving it the extra special care that it required, I tried to ignore these weaknesses and live like everyone else seemed to live – and more. Everyone knows someone who has a 90-year-old relative that is still smoking 40 cigarettes a day, or a friend who can drink ten pints every night and never have a hangover or a business colleague who works 20-hour days and thrives on stress, but such people are freaks of nature, which is why we are always so keen to quote them. It is no surprise to me now that my body packed up, because I now understand what its requirements are. Knowing those requirements and meeting them has given me good health – and if I can do it, so can you.

Warning Signs

All negative symptoms, physical or mental, stem from an imbalance. For example, mood swings are caused by a chemical imbalance, while muscular pain usually results from a structural imbalance. Negative symptoms are there as a warning sign to tell you that your body is not functioning effectively and you need to act before the imbalance becomes unmanageable. If you run your body the way it likes to be run and give it the resources it needs the rewards will be great. If the system works well then the feedback will be positive – plenty of energy, emotional stability and fewer aches and pains.

Of course it is not always just your lifestyle that makes you ill. Any trauma that weakens the body – such as an accident, disease, virus or emotional distress – can be the main trigger for ill health or emotional instability. Exposure to such things is part and parcel of living, which is why you have an inbuilt coping mechanism to deal with them. It is your ability to recover that dictates the state of your health; it is also the deciding factor in whether or not a problem develops. Negative aspects of your lifestyle, such as a bad diet or too much stress, may not be the initial reason for ill health but they can certainly prevent you from recovering. Anything, no matter how small, that puts strain on an already-weakened body will only add to the problem and slow down or even stop the process of recovery.

What Warning Signs Are You Experiencing?

Some physical warning signs:

fatigue
aches and pains
sickness
headaches
dry skin and rashes
food cravings
weight imbalances
a need for stimulants
poor sleep

Some psychological warning signs:

unhappiness
anxiety
disinterest
over-sensitivity
panic attacks
mood swings
feelings of isolation

You Are Unique

Biologically, our bodies should all run in the same way. However, we each have a unique genetic make up, circumstances, environments and individual strengths and weaknesses that dictate how our own body will run. This is precisely why you need to find out what works for you, *personally*. The standard rules of operation should apply – this is why it is so important for you to understand them – but these need to be adapted to suit your own requirements if you want to achieve maximum control over your own health and well-being.

This book can help you find your own route to recovery but, as an individual, you are the only one that can implement change. You are the only one that can discover exactly what works for you from all the information and advice you gather. I uncovered my route to recovery by questioning and experimenting with all the advice I received. It is this same process of discovery that you need to undertake. Conventional routes do not always apply but what does help is knowing how you can make your route to recovery as safe and simple as possible. This book will give you information, options and support to make it an easier process but only you can utilize what you learn to make your own life healthier and happier. If you feel that nothing is worth trying, you won't get very far.

If what you are currently doing is not working, even if it appears to work for many others, you need to find a new approach.

If you are stuck in a rut with a chronic health condition, such as fatigue, you need to look at what is causing and maintaining it. If you don't know this, then you need a bit of knowledge about your body – a bit of body intelligence – because to make a difference you need to know why your body is saying no.

The Perfect Balance

If there is one thing that the body really hates it is extremes of anything for too long. That doesn't mean, however, that you should want or expect a life devoid of difficult situations. Unexpected, scary and challenging events are a natural part of living and we deliberately experiment and take risks in the hope of achieving satisfaction. The body has a system to deal with the ups and downs of living, one that enables it to maintain, or return to, a healthy balance. The body utilizes pairs of opposites to work together – for example, chemicals, responses, muscles – to enable controlled actions to occur throughout the body.

The easiest way of demonstrating this is if you look at a muscular movement. Any movement involves pairs of muscles working together but doing opposite jobs. For example, a simple act like lifting your hand to your mouth will involve one set of muscles contracting while the opposite set relaxes to enable them to expand. This system allows the contracting muscles to bend the arm while the relaxing muscles control its speed and position so that you don't end up hitting yourself in the face. It also allows you to reverse the movement by instigating the opposite response. The body uses various systems of pairing to enable it to cope with continuing changes to your external environment, such as temperature fluctuations, and to deal with the constant changing demands of the internal environment, for example balancing blood sugar as resources are used up and replaced.

This is what is meant by maintaining a healthy balance. The body is equipped to deal with the constant fluctuations of living. Any short-term or one-off fluctuation is generally not a problem if the body is in good health and has plenty of resources – it can then do its job and restore equilibrium. What does affect the health of the body is an extreme imbalance that is not matched by an effective recovery programme, an ongoing imbalance that has no resolution or an action that pushes the body continually into the same sort of imbalance.

Let's look at the actions of two key minerals, potassium and sodium, as an example of how the body maintains balance. These minerals control, amongst other things, fluid balance. Potassium acts as a diuretic that drains excess fluid out of the system and sodium retains fluid to prevent the body becoming dehydrated. This is an ideal pairing system as levels of fluid in the body are fluctuating all the time and need constant readjustment. It also acts as a safety mechanism if the body suffers an injury that results in an excess or loss of fluid, preventing it from further damage and enabling it to recover. If there is an excess or deficiency of either mineral then the healthy balance between the two is lost and the body will begin to develop health problems, such as dehydration or excessive fluid retention, as a result of fluid imbalance.

Much of our misunderstanding of what is and isn't good for us stems from ignorance of the body's need for balance. Everything you do has the potential to harm the body, even if you perceive it as healthy. Too much exercise or too much fruit can be harmful, while chocolate and alcohol can have beneficial qualities if consumed in moderation. It is all a question of balance. This same misunderstanding surfaces when we look at our love-hate relationship with stress.

Stressed Out On Stress

Just mention the word stress and everyone seems to start moaning about how hard it is to cope while, at the same time, they're merrily signing themselves up for things that will generate even more stress in their lives. So why do we have this dilemma with stress where it appears we can't live with it, can't live without it?

It all comes down to our understanding – or, more commonly, misunderstanding – of the meaning of stress. The word stress means a mental, emotional or physical strain or, in terms of physics, a force that produces deformation or strain. When we talk about the negative effects of stress we are referring to doing the same action to excess or for too long, which upsets the body's natural balance to the extent that it reduces its ability to cope with the stresses and strains of living. This reduced ability means that your body will find it harder to restore a healthy balance and this then leads to even greater stress and strain on your system. This can relate to anything you do or don't do – for example, too many hours at work and not enough rest leads to exhaustion, too many pies and not enough activity leads to weight gain and too little excitement and not enough fun leads to unhappiness. All these examples induce stress and it is this stress that leads to a negative result. Stress is a negative sign that the natural healthy balance of the body has been affected. Negative symptoms generated by stress, such as pain and fatigue, are there to warn you that the body is struggling to cope and you need to do something to restore the balance before it gets any worse.

The confusion over our relationship with stress often arises because we confuse negative stress with what is known as the stress response. A healthy body is well equipped to deal with the everyday stresses of living because our lives and our environment are constantly changing and challenging us, so stress is bound to occur in some form or another on a daily basis. The body deals with this through the stress response – a natural, biological response designed to enable your body to do all the things you demand of it to keep you alive and happy. Stress is an unhealthy and excessive amount of pressure that leads to harm, whereas the stress response is, without sounding too dramatic, the thing that keeps you living. Without it you would quite literally not get out of bed in the morning. It is meant to be used and you thrive off the positive stimulation it can generate. In fact, many people suffer from the symptoms of stress because they are under-stimulated and have little pleasure as a result of not using their stress response enough. To live a happy and healthy life you need to activate your stress response and make it work for you so that you can achieve, survive and experience pleasure from stimulation.

The problem with activating the stress response is that, in the process of using it, you generate wear and tear on the body and drain resources. Of course, this is the whole reason why you need to provide resources in the first place – to power the body and keep it in good repair. It is a simple process of having the right equipment and resources to carry out a job, doing that job and then replacing resources when you have finished so that you can then go on and do another job. In terms of the stress response, the body's balancing agent is relaxation. Your stress response stimulates your body to enable it to act but to keep it in good working order your body needs an opposite response that counter-balances the effects of the stress response. This is the purpose of relaxation.

Rejuvenating Relaxation

The stress response is your problem solver. It will only be triggered if you have a problem or set it a task to do. Its only purpose is to resolve the situation as quickly and as effectively as possible, irrespective of the toll that takes on the body. This is because, in theory, once the task is complete, the relaxation response will take over and clean up the mess, repair the damage and replace the used resources. This is why we have to sleep every night – to repair the damage incurred by the body during the day and to process new resources, such as a fresh energy supply, to replace those used up during our waking hours. A healthy body should wake up refreshed in the morning and will be tired by the end of a stimulating day because energy supplies have been used and wear and tear has been incurred. Your body switches you off at the end of the day so that it can concentrate on restoration, recovery and regeneration, thus enabling you to go out and live life to the full the next day. If you wake up feeling exhausted, have dramatic energy slumps through the day, have consistently low energy levels or find it hard to sleep, this is a sign that your body is not running effectively. If this applies to you, your first step is to look at the balance between stimulation and relaxation in your life, because too much of either for too long will have a detrimental effect on your health.

How Relaxed Are You?

- Do you claim that it is impossible for you to relax because of your busy life?
  You may feel that taking time to relax is a frivolous, self-indulgent thing that cannot be fitted into your hectic life. However, if you want to lead a stimulating and satisfying life, you will need to make time for relaxation.
- Do you feel tired all the time?
  You may once have had a busy life but are being forced to slow down because of the state of your energy levels and overall health. However, this does not mean you are necessarily more relaxed. Your reduced capabilities could be making you anxious and frustrated and, as a result, your body finds it hard to switch off.

- Do you wake up feeling extremely tired?
  If your body is exhausted it will sleep but you may not be experiencing a deep relaxing sleep if you are creating more wear and tear during the day than your body can put right during the night. In addition, an inability to switch off anxiety will result in low energy levels.
- Do you feel you should always be doing something even when you are not?
  Even when you are not physically moving you could still be over-stressing the body with constant anxiety, thinking about what you should or want to be doing. In fact, lack of positive mental stimulation or physical activity is one of the biggest causes of stress.
- When you are tired do you reach for a quick fix?
  Low energy levels and an inability to relax can be generated by diet. Stimulants, a poor diet or a diet high in sugar and fat will induce stimulation. You may think you are relaxing with a glass of wine and a cigarette but in fact you are stimulating your system when all it wants to do is relax.
- Do you suffer from constant health problems?
  Stress is not just something that affects the mind, it can have a detrimental effect on any part of the body. If your body is not getting the 'downtime' it needs to maintain health and energy levels then problems can surface anywhere in the body, irrespective of the source of the original stress.

Time To Switch Off

The stress response will only switch off when it feels it is safe to do so; when all the problems and tasks that you have set it have been resolved or when you stop supplying it with stimulants such as coffee and alcohol. Difficulty in relaxing can be the result of emotional insecurities, anxieties, lifestyle habits or an on-going problem with your physical health. This is because your body will not switch off the stress response while it has a problem to resolve. Unfortunately, if you do not relax then your body will be unable to keep up with its day-to-day maintenance and a backlog of jobs will build up. The combination of this and the additional pressure from the initial problem makes it even harder for the body to cope. Not surprisingly, if you find it hard to relax or have trouble sleeping you are bound to feel awful because the body has been unable to restore your energy levels – and the more awful you feel, the less capable your body is of resolving your problem, because it is finding it hard to function properly.

I can now hear you screaming, 'So how can you switch off when life makes it so difficult to do so?' Life is about dealing with multiple issues at once, some small, but on-going, and some large and unexpected. You cannot remove stress from your life, and often you don't want to, it is more a case of dealing with it effectively so that you get the maximum benefit from living with minimum damage to your system. The body has mechanisms to stimulate and relax but it also needs the right emotional responses to initiate these mechanisms.

You can mechanically switch off your stress response anywhere by:

- Deep breathing – just four or five deep breaths can be enough to switch off stress, so incorporate regular deep breathing breaks into your day.
- Relaxing your muscles – pick out a tense muscle and focus your mind on relaxing it.
- Massage – apply gentle pressure to your skin with your fingertips in small, circular movements on your hands, forehead, scalp, feet or shoulders.

You can create the right emotional atmosphere by:

- Registering to return to a task – write down what is worrying you or needs to be done and to give your body a breathing space arrange to come back to it tomorrow, next week, in an hour or in five minutes.
- Focus on something soothing – take a few minutes to think about a relaxing environment like a hot sandy beach or clouds moving in a bright blue sky.
- Find something to make you smile – watch a comedy, play with the children, run through the park or just sit back, stretch and make a big grin on your face.

Benefit From Pleasure

Achieving a healthy balance between stimulation and relaxation is vital. We need to use our stress response, but, in order to keep the body fully functional, we also need a system to deal with the effects of implementing the stress response. So, you may be wondering, why use the stress response if it creates so much damage?

One of the most fundamental requirements of the body is to experience pleasure and satisfaction. These are the positive responses that tell you that life is worth living and you are living it well. You will get negative signs when your body is unhappy but you will also get positive responses when it is happy with what you are doing. These signs are there to tell you what will and won't improve your chances of a happy, healthy life. Your positive stimuli come from chemical and hormonal responses. These are the so-called 'happy drugs', such as endorphins and serotonin, that give you your motivation for living. They are released during stimulation, not only to help achieve the task in hand but also in recognition of a job done well and as an incentive to continue taking risks and trying to achieve. In order to experience this we need to instigate the stress response. As I have said before, many people suffer from health problems such as depression, fatigue and anxiety because they are under-stimulated and are therefore not getting their daily dose of nature's happy drugs.

Quick Ways To Get A Happy Fix

- Look at all the things that didn't go wrong today.
- Focus on how well you coped with all the things that did go wrong today.
- Make an effort to smile even if you don't feel like it.
- Call someone you love and tell them so.
- Say thank you and mean it.
- Do something constructive about a task you have been putting off.
- Stand and sit up straight, don't slump.
- Pamper yourself, even if it's just a scented bath or a DIY manicure.

You may think these things are stupid, pointless and won't help because you are far too unwell, but every little helps. If you are tired, run down, fed up or feel unwell then you are more likely to be unhappy – but happiness is one of the best cure-all drugs naturally and freely available. Feeling better about yourself, your life and your situation is the first step to improving your lot. If you give your body time out to relax and have fun it will be physically more capable of coping with the unpleasant aspects of your life. Your body will say no to negative stress but yes to relaxation, and it loves positive stimulation. Get the balance right and your body will work for you and not against you.

Body Operations

Although the body is extremely complex it does have a very simplistic system of operation. It has specific benchmark levels, such as perfect body temperature, blood pressure or blood sugar, but it does not expect or necessarily want to be stuck at these all the time. It likes variety and taking calculated risks because it likes to progress. It is not just a case of finding a healthy balance but knowing how to maintain and improve it so that the body never gets bored or under-stimulated. A healthy balance comes from knowing how to deal with imbalances rather than trying to create a stress-free life.

The body is a physical system that is designed to deal with your mental requirements. Your body needs to be able to solve a whole variety of problems and perform tasks, all of which involves physical effort. The natural balancing system that your body operates under is able to deal effectively with all this physical and mental effort and keep itself in good health – but it relies on your ability to operate it correctly. To achieve optimum health, the body likes to be run in the way it was designed to be run – through a balance of stimulation and relaxation. To enable this balance to operate you also need to supply your body with adequate resources, such as essential nutrients and water, to power it. If resources are low and the balance is upset then your body will struggle to cope. This is often when we resort to quick fixes to keep us going in the short term. Unfortunately, in the long term, these actually drain your resources even further, resulting in more stress and strain on your body.

Quick Fixes That Unbalance The Body

Smoking – each cigarette smoked can reduce oxygen input by half for up to two hours
Alcohol – can prevent the absorption of essential nutrients

Foods high in sugar or fat – unbalances blood glucose levels, affecting mood and energy levels
Processed foods – often low in nutrients and full of additives, straining the digestive system
High salt foods – causes fluid retention and pushes up blood pressure
Caffeine – dehydrates the body and increases toxicity

An addiction or constant craving for these quick fixes is a sign that your body is out of balance. All these things may become a compulsion for someone with an imbalanced body because they are all things that will give them a temporary energy boost and a quick pleasure fix – which is why we like them so much when we are tired and fed up. Unfortunately, they also heap additional strain and stress on an already run-down system, reducing energy levels further and preventing the body from running effectively.

Adrenaline Rush

The key chemical that kick-starts the stress response is adrenaline. Its role is to put the body on red alert and flood it with as much energy as possible to achieve maximum strength and brainpower. It is this effect that makes adrenaline so appealing – because that rush of energy makes you feel fantastic. In a split second adrenaline brings in huge amounts of oxygen by changing the way you breathe and by diverting existing energy supplies from elsewhere in the body. Adrenaline works to deadlines: the more immediate the deadline, the greater its ability to get the body moving and thinking. This is a good thing – in fact, it is a great thing because it can get you out of danger fast. However, adrenaline is only designed to be released in short, sharp doses. There is nothing wrong with putting your body on maximum output but the longer the output of adrenaline is sustained, or the more regularly it occurs, the greater the wear and tear on your body and the faster the drain on energy supplies. High levels of stimulation require high levels of body maintenance and energy production, and too much stimulation for too long, without a break, is unsustainable.

The stress response is designed to run to a time scale. Get the benefit, solve the problem, finish the task, get the reward and then stop to restore and refresh. Adrenaline is there at the start of a stress response to help you make a fast decision on the best way to act. Therefore, in order to work with the stress response, decisions need to be made quickly. A good deal of stress and anxiety is the result of indecision. If your body is unable to switch off your stress response because you are unable to decide how to resolve the problem, then your energy resources will run very low.

If you have a problem making decisions it is useful to recognize that deciding not to act or postponing the action is still a decision. If weighing up a decision is making you unhappy or causing you anxiety and stress, you need to take time out to relax. Switching off the stress response, even momentarily, will give your body time to rejuvenate energy supplies and calm your mind to help you see the problem more rationally. When you reactivate your stress response, a fresh flow of adrenaline will help you act with greater effect.

Every Breath You Take

If you think about what adrenaline needs to do to get the body physically moving, it is not difficult to understand why this quickly uses up your supplies of energy. For a start, it changes the way you breathe. Breathing regulates the amount of oxygen taken into the body and as oxygen is a major component of energy, more will be needed to enable adrenaline to do its job. Adrenaline requires a huge amount of energy to enable it to increase energy levels dramatically, so it changes your breathing to short and shallow. This allows the lungs to bring in a large amount of oxygen in a very short space of time but it also means that huge amounts of available resources have been used in the process and, as these resources run out, the body starts to tire. You need energy to utilize more energy therefore an increase in energy output will use up existing resources much more quickly.

Think about how you feel when you do anything that involves an additional amount of effort, like running for instance. Your body will utilize all the available energy to increase your capacity to go faster but this means that it will tire much more rapidly than if you walked the same distance, because the energy supply will run out much more quickly. Your body is capable of running at this speed, you just need to remember that it involves more effort; in fact the benefit of running fast is that you will release more pleasure responses so there is a greater feel-good factor. When you stop running, or are forced to stop because of fatigue, you will be panting for breath because the effort involved in short, shallow breathing and the speed at which you used up your resources has resulted in reduced energy levels. This means that your body cannot continue bringing in the high levels of oxygen required to keep you stimulated so intake becomes dramatically reduced, resulting in a further drop in energy. If you do not give your body time to recover, your energy levels will continue to fall because your body cannot keep up with production. Consistently low energy means your body cannot run itself effectively and, as a result, it will find it hard to produce new energy supplies, leaving you feeling tired all the time.

An Example

The body only has a limited amount of fuel available at any one time and as it burns fuel it needs replacement energy supplies. A camping stove provides a good analogy – it has a container of heat-producing fuel to enable it to work, just as your body has energy supplies available to give you power. If you burn the cooker flame on a low heat then the fuel supply will probably last all day but the heat will not be that great. However, if you cook something on a high flame the fuel will run out a lot quicker. You can use this higher flame as much as you like – but only if you are prepared to put in the additional maintenance and investment. On a high flame the fuel canister will continuously need changing and the cooker will incur more damage, therefore it will need more of your time and effort to keep it in good working order. Your body is no different. However, while you can simply buy a new stove when you've worn the old one out, you can't trade in your worn-out body for a new one.

What you therefore have to decide is how much you can demand of it, given how much effort you are prepared to put in to maintain it. Frustration and anxiety emerge when the user expects maximum performance without understanding the full extent of what is required to sustain this performance, or is unwilling to invest the effort involved in high maintenance.

How Are You Running Your Body?

Do you often work late?
Do you get constantly impatient or frustrated when things slow you down?
Do you make long lists of things to do but never seem to get much done?
Do you only ever stop because you are forced to by fatigue?
Do you never have enough hours in the day?
Are you always late?
Do you eat on the run, have irregular eating patterns or eat a lot of ready meals?
Do you smoke?
Do you drink alcohol more than four times a week?
Do you flake out in front of the television every night?
Do you never seem to have enough energy to get motivated?

If you do any of these things regularly then there is a good chance that your body is not running effectively. Your body needs to be either relaxed or stimulated and learning to differentiate between the two will help you restore and maintain a healthy balance.

Make The Break

When your body is relaxed it will use a completely different method of breathing from that experienced during periods of stimulation. The relaxation response utilizes long, deep breaths to counterbalance the short, shallow breaths of the stress response. This enables the body to rebalance the intake of oxygen to a normal, sustainable level. It is important that this balance is continuously assessed as sustained periods of either stress or under-stimulation can result in low energy levels, health problems and emotional instability. We have seen how stimulation physically exhausts the body, however, if you have continuously low activity levels, or little mental stimulation, the body will start to shut down as it sees no reason to produce energy that you are clearly not using. This will make you feel lethargic and de-motivated, so you can see why it is so important to keep the responses moving regularly from one to the other. Prolonged periods of stimulation or anxiety produce high levels of fatigue due to a loss of energy resources and excess wear and tear on the body, while prolonged periods of under-stimulation and inactivity generate fatigue as it sets your metabolism at a low tick-over and deprives you of pleasure stimuli.

The greater and more prolonged the stress response, the greater the need to utilize the relaxation response, as they work together as a team. Greater stimulation can easily result in more fatigue if your body does not get an opportunity to restore and replenish. Long periods of excessive stimulation will mean your body will need to rest for longer to recover, so creating breaks in your stress responses will help to sustain energy levels and speed up the recovery process. On the other hand, if your body is under-stimulated for prolonged periods you will have low energy output and little motivation and pleasure. Hopefully you can now see how easy it is to upset the balance but, similarly, how straightforward restoring and maintaining the balance can be. This is why it is important to listen to what your body is telling you. Negative symptoms may be unpleasant but learning to understand what they are trying to tell you is vital if you want to feel good.

Are You Low On Energy?

If so, then ask yourself why:

- Is it because you are living life to the full, working hard, playing hard and love your quick-fix stimulants?
  Then you need to incorporate relaxation and a healthier attitude to what you put into your body if you want to keep going at a fast pace. Greater levels of stimulation are rewarding but they require much more care and maintenance.
- Is it because you never have time to stop and have lots of negative stress?
  Then you need to incorporate relaxation into your schedule and introduce more positive stimulation into your life if you want to feel good.
- Is it because you are unhappy and frustrated with your life?
  Then you definitely need positive stimulation but you also need to address those pent-up anxieties that are stressing your body out.

Of course you could be low on energy due to all three of the above. This is why it is so important to assess your own personal situation – because there will be a combination of reasons behind your problems that will be specific to you.

Stress does not just happen as a result of overdoing things, it also relates to what you eat, how happy you are, how much you achieve, any illnesses or physical weaknesses that you have and how active you are. Remember, being inactive does not mean you are relaxed; many people are anxious and frustrated about being inactive. Similarly, you may be doing things that you think will relax you, like smoking or having a cup of tea, but again you are stressing your body even more because these things act as stimulants. Learn to make the distinction between relaxation and stimulation by becoming more aware of how you feel. Monitor your responses to make sure you do not get stuck at either end of the scale for too long because too much of anything for too long is all your body needs to say no.

Stages Of Stress

So we have established that adrenaline is great in small, swift doses but force your body to prolong production and you will just wear it out. The other dominant effect that adrenaline has on the health of your body is through its ability to divert resources from one area of the body to supply another. When the stress response is triggered, the priority of adrenaline is to supply the brain and muscles with as much energy and resources as possible to make you as strong and as quick-thinking as possible. Obviously in a life-threatening situation there is not much that internal systems like your digestive system, renal system and skin can do to help, therefore energy supplies and resources are diverted away from the body systems that have no value in completing the immediate task in hand. The most obvious example of this is when someone who is over-excited or afraid goes 'white as a ghost'. This occurs because adrenaline diverts the blood supply away from the skin, resulting in a loss of skin colour.

Basically the stress response can upset the natural balance of the body to enable it to deal with immediate problems because they could be life threatening. The body will therefore do everything it can to utilize every resource available, with little concern as to what effect this will have on its long-term health and well-being. This means that prolonged stress and anxiety could result in whole areas of your body being deprived of the essential resources they need to maintain healthy operations. This is why the symptoms of stress are so diverse, because it can have an effect on every part of your body. The stress response is designed to deliberately upset the natural healthy balancing systems of the body to enable it to get the job done. Short term this is not a problem, because once the threat is removed, normal functioning is restored, but long term, believe me, it takes its toll.

One Small Imbalance

If you look at all your body functions and the components required to enable them to operate, it is clear just how interconnected the various functions of the body are. I have already mentioned the balancing act between potassium and sodium. These two minerals work together on a variety of functions, including maintaining internal fluid levels and nerve responses. When the stress response is activated, adrenaline will get rid of any available potassium and retain as much sodium as possible in order to raise the blood pressure. Higher blood pressure increases energy levels and a simple way of raising your blood pressure is by increasing internal fluid capacity. In the short term this is fine; in fact it is great, as you will feel much more alert and full of energy. Long term, an excess of sodium with the absence of potassium leads to fluid retention. A fluid imbalance will affect not just your heart and kidneys but disrupt all your body systems in one way or another – as well as blowing you up like a balloon. An imbalance of these two minerals means that other functions regulated by potassium and sodium are also disrupted. Nerve responses will become dysfunctional, causing you to overreact to pain and emotions, or experience sensations of numbness and disinterest. As all minerals interrelate, an excess or deficiency in one will have a knock-on effect on all your bodily processes, for instance muscle function and energy production. It is obvious then how one small but prolonged imbalance can start to have an overall effect on the health of the body. Now imagine the whole range of minerals, vitamins and nutrients required to run your body, the functions that need to occur and the systems that need to operate – a small imbalance in each of these areas can add up to one big imbalance.

Small Symptoms To Look Out For

Hot flushes and cold sweats
Hyperactivity and sudden waves of fatigue
Pins and needles and sensitive skin
Loss of feeling and over-sensitivity
Sudden emotional reactions and complete disinterest
Overactive mind and brain fog
Insomnia at night and intense tiredness during the day

Remember we are looking at an imbalance, so symptoms will often swing from one extreme to another. Alternatively, you may suffer from one extreme symptom but it is unlikely that it will be in isolation. Multiple small but chronic symptoms are signs that your body is finding it hard to cope with whatever stresses and strains it is under. Your symptoms may no longer be small or minor but it is likely that they would have started out this way, perhaps years earlier. This could well be the point at which your imbalance started and this is where you will find your first clues to recovery. The World Health Organization says that good health isn't just the absence of illness but the presence of optimum emotional and physical well-being. When did you start to lose yours?

Time To Act

To keep your body functioning effectively you need to...

- Experience a combination of positive stimulation and relaxation
- Supply your body with the right resources
- Keep your stress response short by breaking it up

To keep your stress responses healthy you need to...

- Feel confident in your capabilities
- Have a good incentive
- Make a quick decision

The next step to a healthy stress response is to act immediately on that quick decision. So much stress and anxiety is generated by not acting to accomplish a need or desire. In all the various stages of the stress response, the body flushes a variety of activating responses and hormones through the body. Initially the main ones are adrenaline and cortisol, because they are designed to get things moving. Once a decision to act has been made a new supply of chemicals and responses, designed specifically to help you deal with action, flood into the system. This is why it is important to keep the system moving, as the body needs to be continuously topped up with the appropriate supplies. Like the food in your fridge, these supplies get used up and can go off. The term 'bottled up' is very appropriate because in this state your body is like a shaken champagne bottle desperate to pop its cork. In the body, frustration, anxiety and anger start to build up if all this ready-prepared energy is not utilized. This additional pressure will put a huge strain on your body if it is left to build over an extended period. Eventually this pressure will either erupt as an emotional outburst or just loose its fizz, leaving you feeling exhausted but your problem remains unresolved. The continuing anxiety of this situation puts a further strain on your body, making it even harder for you to resolve the issue. This vicious circle must be addressed if you want to get your body to work well for you.

The Cycle Of Stress

So you have an incentive, you decide on your plan of action and act on it; now it is time to collect your reward. This is the point when you need to assess if your actions have been effective or not and this is where those wonderful happy drugs kick in. Even difficult, scary or unpleasant actions need to be assessed in a positive manner if you want to keep your stress responses healthy. If things have gone badly then time to reflect is vital to enable you to recognize the benefit of any given situation. Even if the results are bad, if you can prove that you have learnt from the experience or can demonstrate that a new course of action can improve on the situation, then you will receive positive feedback. This is the time when your body needs to rest and reflect and this is all part of your continuing cycle of survival. If your body is given time to restore itself then you will be more than capable of continuing to improve your life. Once your body is rested, a new incentive to improve your situation will result in a surge of energy as your stress response is triggered. To keep the energy flowing you need to keep the cycle going from decision, to action, result assessment, receiving your reward and then giving your body time out to rest so that it can keep this cycle going continuously.

It is often our attitudes or expectations that prevent us from bringing a stress response to an end – but it is vitally important for the body to experience a cut-off point. The body needs to have a purpose for all that hard work, and feelings of pleasure or satisfaction give it that. You cannot experience results if you never draw things to a conclusion, therefore ongoing stresses will never produce those feel-good feelings your body so desperately craves.

The Healthy Cycle

INCENTIVE – DECISION – ACTION – RESULT – ASSESSMENT – REWARD – REST

If you look back at prehistoric times, it is clear that survival was a much more immediate concern. If you were a caveman being chased by a big carnivorous animal then it wasn't hard to find an incentive, make a decision, act and – assuming you managed to get back to your cave – relax. The stress response may seem more in tune with those primeval demands than the ones you have in your world but those who survive successfully today are the ones who run with the natural system. Indecisive or inactive cavemen didn't live for very long and although you may not be faced with predators on a regular basis, you still have to run your body effectively in order to have a healthy life. When clients come to me and say 'I feel ill and want to be healthy but don't expect me to give this up or stop doing that', I point out that it is their choice. They can either carry on as they are and feel unhealthy and unhappy or they make changes that will make them feel better. If someone wants to carry on running around like a headless chicken on a poor diet with no rest up, continue to smoke or refuse to confront their emotional issues, then that's fine, but they can't expect anything to change. Ultimately, it is how you use or abuse your system that dictates how good you feel physically and how well you cope mentally – this is not necessarily something that is dictated by the difficulty of the situation you are in.

Go Back In Time

Take yourself back to prehistoric times and imagine you are sunbathing outside your cave when a great big scary animal appears out of the blue. Immediately your stress response is activated and your body is flooded with adrenaline. First you need to make a very quick decision about what you intend to do and then you need physical strength to enable you to act. The stress response is often referred to as the 'fight or flight' response because basically these are the two usual options available to anyone in a threatening situation. Once you have done either of these things and are, hopefully, out of danger, you will need to rest. Now that the immediate threat is over your body will bring in negative symptoms like pain and fatigue to give you an indication of how much time you need to rest and what repair work needs to be done. Even though the injury and the drain on resources happened during the stress response your body didn't want to bring it to your attention at that point because it could have distracted you from saving yourself. We have all heard of people who have had a heart attack the week they retired or perhaps you always go down with a bug at the start of every holiday. This can be the result of the stress response deliberately masking problems until it knows that the body is safe. Once you relax, a whole batch of negative issues can suddenly surface and, not surprisingly, this reaction can make you less likely to relax in the future. The longer you keep a stress going, the more you will fear stopping.

Just before I was ill, I was running on turbo drive and thought it was fantastic. I told everyone I thrived on stress and felt ill and washed out if I ever took time off. When I did have a day off, all I wanted to do was sleep and I felt awful, so I kept going. Eventually my body got to a point where it could cope no longer and just packed up. Unfortunately, I associated fatigue with being idle so all I wanted to do was get moving again. Even though I could hardly move, I still tried to force my body and mind to keep going because I thought it just needed a bit of a kick. Even though my exhaustion meant all I could do was lie around all day, I was never relaxed because I was constantly anxious about what I should or would like to be doing. Accepting that my body needed to rest, and making it as comfortable and pleasurable as possible, was a big turning point in my recovery. Once I started to work with my body, my body started to respond in a positive way because I was giving it an opportunity to work in the way it wanted to work and providing it with the things it needed to work.

Remember, stress is a part of living and has to be accepted as such – it is how you deal with it that dictates whether its effects will be detrimental or not.

Messing About With Emotions

When you are tired does it make you emotionally sensitive?
Do you regularly get angry or frustrated?
Do you often burst into tears for no apparent reason?
When you are unhappy are you more sensitive to pain?
Do you associate happiness with being full of energy?

Emotional and physical body responses are all intertwined so it is not surprising that the state of your health has a huge influence on your state of mind and vice versa. If you have emotional problems then doing everything you can to improve your health will make those emotional issues easier to resolve. Similarly, an ongoing emotional issue can trigger physical health problems therefore your attitude can play a big part in any programme of self-help health care.

So far we have looked at the physical effects of stress but your emotional reaction to a situation has a huge influence on the outcome. Put yourself back in the caveman's situation again and imagine you are at the point of fight or flight. If you choose to fight and in the process incur an injury but survive, or if you choose to run back to the cave and get teased for being a coward, then you could feel disappointment and a sense of failure, even though you managed to deal with the problem successfully. The pain or criticism you received could then prevent you from going outside again because of fear of further pain or humiliation should there be another animal attack. However, it is not the animal that is stopping you from enjoying your life, because you have proved that you can deal with it, it is the pain or humiliation you experienced because of it. This fear will now limit your life and make it a more anxious and less enjoyable existence. Your lack of activity and achievement as a result of your experience will destabilize your emotional state and your fear will intensify as your under-stimulated imagination begins to visualize even scarier animals – or even ones that can get into caves. These anxieties will drain your energy levels and the lack of positive stimulation will result in more unhappiness. The negative emotional input from this event has prevented you from running your responses through the natural effective cycle. Constant anxiety due to inactivity and indecision is preventing you from experiencing positive feedback and the pleasures of energy rushes from stimulation, as well as depriving your body of relaxation, and this gives you little incentive to change your situation. However, it is not the result or the situation that has lead to this but rather your attitude towards it.

If you had taken a different approach then the emotional feedback could have been very different. For example, if you had asked for help from your friends in the cave you would have been less likely to get hurt or criticized and, even if you were, you could accept this as a negative consequence of achieving overall success. However, the emotional feedback could also be made more positive simply by seeing the event from a rational point of view rather than a personal one. For example, if you are going to take on big scary animals then obviously there is a risk of injury, and if others are scathing about your successful escape then it may simply be because it brings to light their own inadequacies. Having rationalized the outcome you could then move on from the event, perhaps feeling inspired to do something constructive about the threat, like putting up a fence or digging a trench. Such a positive and constructive approach to life and the problems it throws up fits in with the way the body likes to be run and gives it a much better chance of maintaining energy levels and remaining happy and healthy.

The balance that is indicative of good health comes from keeping your body active and stimulated, giving it time to repair and recover and keeping your attitudes and approaches to living rational and positive. Without this sort of balance your body will find it hard to do anything.

Look At How You Run Your System

Do you find it hard to get motivated?
Do you find it hard to make a decision?
Do you get anxious when you need to act?
Do you suffer from constant disappointment?
Do you feel stuck in a rut?
Do you experience a lack of pleasure and satisfaction?
Do you suffer from constant anxiety?

If you answer yes to any of these then your body is not operating effectively and you could well be experiencing stress as a result. In part two we'll look at ways to deal with emotional issues but first you need to determine what type of stress you suffer from.

Are You Active Or Passive? Stress Chart

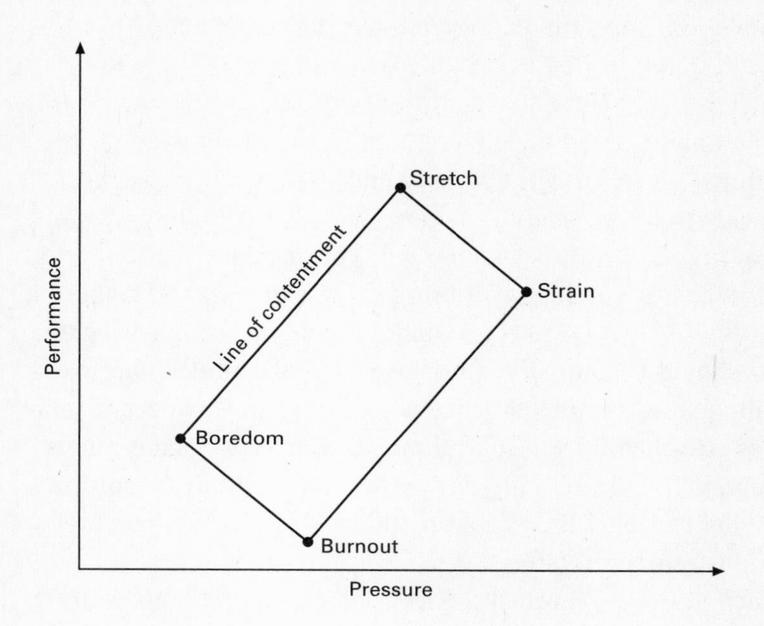

To combat stress you first need to determine if you are suffering from active or passive stress. Take a look at the chart – we'll start with boredom. If you have very little pressure in your life, you will under-perform, which leads to boredom, leading to a reduced output of positive stimuli that could result in general unhappiness and dissatisfaction. If this applies to you, then you are suffering from passive stress.

If you increase the amount of pressure in your life and stretch your abilities, your performance will increase, producing greater satisfaction and interest. I call the line between the states of boredom and stretching your abilities, the line of contentment. A happy and fulfilling life is one that moves up and down between these two states but stays well within the range. It would be nice to put a dot in the middle and say that is where I want to be but, if you were there all the time, I am sure you would get bored with it! Your circumstances, environment and your need to improve life will mean that you can never be in a static state, however, you need to be constantly monitoring your position on this line to make sure you are not stuck at one extreme state for too long. If you have a healthy body it will naturally try to steer a course between these two states – if you are bored it will want to go out and get stimulated; conversely, if you are over-stretching yourself it will naturally encourage you to ease up.

If you stretch yourself to achieve success then although your level of pressure will rise, so too will your performance, therefore the extra effort will bring satisfying rewards, making it all worthwhile. As you become more accomplished, any negative effects should be short-lived because as your abilities improve the initial strain of inexperience will disappear. However, if your body is stretched for too long through an excess of continuous pressure, you will tire and your performance will drop, putting you under strain. If this scenario applies to you, then you are suffering from active stress.

When you have reached the level of strain, although your performance will be falling, your pressures will be growing because it will be taking you longer to do things. The onset of fatigue will reduce your ability to perform and this will, in turn, add to the problem because you are more likely to make mistakes that will create more pressure. This is how the body spirals into stress problems. You are tired and less capable and because of that you create more problems. Things take longer to do and you achieve less, which then makes you feel unhappy and dissatisfied. You will burn out when this level of strain becomes too much for your body to bear. The downward spiral that leads to burnout may seem speedy but for most people it takes years of slow health disintegration as energy levels fall, emotional states decline and internal systems start to shut down. On a positive note, this means that if you spot the signs early and understand where they could lead, you have the time to deal with them before they cause too many problems.

If you remain under strain then rising pressures and reduced performance could result in burnout. When you reach this stage, you will be unable to cope and will therefore be forced to reduce the amount you do or stop altogether. Although in this state you may perceive you have loads more pressure, in reality you have reduced your workload down to almost nothing and handed your responsibilities over to someone more capable. This means that you are also under-performing, which will make you feel dissatisfied, frustrated and even more exhausted.

Once you have had time to rest, your health may start to improve and you will start to climb slowly back towards boredom. However, you will now fear that if you push yourself the whole unpleasant process will happen again. As a result, you may well deliberately avoid stimulation for fear of burning out – but this will also deprive you of those wonderful happy drugs and energy rushes that stimulation induces. This dilemma leaves sufferers seemingly trapped in a world where they are under-stimulated and have no energy. Many people I see with chronic fatigue are stuck in that boredom zone because they are living with the constant anxiety and fear of their situation – fear of stimulation, fear caused by not knowing what has happened, fear of it happening again and anxiety about their inability. I know how that feels because I have been all around the chart and got stuck in a few places on it myself.

If you understand how you fit into this pattern, it is easier to see which direction you need to take to improve your situation. Somehow you need to get back onto the line of contentment. If you are suffering from active stress you need a programme of relaxation and repair. If you are suffering from passive stress you need positive stimulation and a programme of energy recovery. Whatever end of the scale you're currently at, you need to stop and begin to move in a new, more positive direction.

How To Bring Back The Balance

1. KEEP THE SYSTEM RUNNING: Remember the order of operation – incentive, decision, action, result assessment, reward and rest. Keep it moving to keep your stress levels healthy. If you make quick decisions and act immediately you will cut down on anxiety and keep your stress responses healthy and satisfying. Remember, your approach and attitude play a big part in how stress affects your health. Reap the benefit from your stress response, not the damage.
2. KEEP THE RESPONSES SEPARATE: You should be either relaxed or stimulated. If your body wants to rest and you are full of anxiety about what you could or should be doing then the body does not know whether it is relaxed and repairing or stimulated and solving. When you need a break, distract your mind with pleasurable thoughts.
3. LEARN TO RELAX: If you find it hard to switch off mentally then remember that you can do it mechanically. There are so many ways to relax but the most effective ones involve deep breathing. You can do it in the bath, on the bus, at work and you can do it in 20 seconds or 20 minutes so there really is no excuse.
4. BREAK UP STRESS: Rather than seeing the whole day as one long dose of stress, break it up into individual, small stress responses and end each one with a mini relaxation break. Look at all the little tasks that take up your day: for example, phone calls, driving, time on the computer, taking the children to school or finishing a work project. Every time you put down the phone, stop at traffic lights or finish a conversation make these natural breaks a time to relax. Just a few deep breaths or a quick stretch will make that break. Don't wait for your energy to fall, take small steps to keep the levels up.
5. HELP YOUR HEALTH: Maintaining good health should not interfere with living, it should be a natural part of it.

Restoring health, on the other hand, will involve time and effort so you need to invest the time initially. Listen to your body, it is always trying to tell you something so learn to read its language. Negative symptoms are there to tell you that something is wrong. Address them at an early stage while they are easier to resolve. Changing your habits to healthy ones should not be seen as dull and boring but as a way of making your life more exciting and stimulating. Believe me, there is nothing more dull and boring than being unhealthy.

6 ENJOY SOME POSITIVE STIMULATION: A healthy, happy body needs stimulation. You need to be able to deal with stressful situations but you also need to experience satisfaction and pleasure. Unfortunately, sad and bad things will always happen in life so focus your energies on making good things happen. Recent research in the US found that one group suffering from depression showed better results from taking two brisk walks a day than another group who were on anti-depressants – so it is possible for you to take control of the way you feel.

Your aim now is to find your own line of contentment. This is where you will get satisfaction from achievement without burning your body out in the process. We cannot expect to feel fantastic all the time and accidents and illnesses will happen, what you want to achieve is control. Good health comes from feeling in control of your body, knowing that you can influence the way you feel and having the ability to recover. Your body is your machine for living. Like any machine, it pays to follow the instructions.

Vital Energy

When you understand how the body produces energy, it becomes easier to see how we become fatigued. We tend to think of energy as something we need to move the parts of the body we can physically control, such as muscles, and to help the brain with our thought processes. Although this is true, a much larger percentage of your daily energy supply is used to run all the systems in the body that you have no control over – for instance, your heart, kidneys and digestive system. The amount of calories your body needs to run all its system is referred to as its resting metabolic rate, or RMR. This refers to what your body requires *before* you can even attempt to do all the things you want to do, like move and think. The average woman, for example, requires approximately 1700 calories a day just to run the internal workings of her body. Therefore, if her calorie intake is around 2500 per day, approximately two thirds of that is used to do the jobs she has no control over. So you can see why your body hates to be put on a low calorie diet – it fears it will not have enough usable energy to go around.

The priority energy supply is used to keep the body ticking over. Whatever is left is then available to be used for conscious actions. If your body is under constant or extreme stress the additional workload and the increase in wear and tear will result in your body needing more energy and resources to operate, leaving less available for your conscious purposes. As more energy is used internally, your movement and thought processes will reduce in strength as energy levels fall, resulting in poor concentration and physical fatigue. It can also cause you to crave stimulants and high-calorie foods in a desperate attempt to boost flagging energy levels – however, the additional strain these generate means that your body has to work even harder, putting it under further stress.

The brain is one of the highest internal energy users so any drop in energy will have a huge effect on your brain's ability to function. Your brain is your control centre; it oversees every movement, response and function. Think of how you feel when you are tired and run down. You find it hard to concentrate, your movements slow down, your emotions are all over the place, you make silly mistakes and you forget things altogether. If low energy has this noticeable effect on your ability to function, just imagine what it is doing to the internal workings of your body. Processes and responses will be affected in the same way. They will slow down through exhaustion, send out wrong information or won't send any out at all, systems will be put on a low tick-over and any repair and maintenance programme will be put on hold while the body frantically diverts what resources it has to immediate priorities and life-maintaining processes. The body needs to supply essential operational systems before your demands are even considered. If energy levels are constantly low then what is available is used to keep the systems of the body operational. This means there is very little remaining for you to use elsewhere.

We do have the ability to store energy and the body's method of doing this – by storing it in fat cells – causes many of us great distress. Most of us have a good supply of stored energy and some of us have an excessive supply, so why do our energy levels fluctuate or remain low when the body has the ability to store a constant and often excessive supply of potential energy? The main reason is that the body finds it hard to convert those supplies into usable energy because it does not have the right resources or processes available to allow it to do so.

Symptoms Of An Energy Imbalance

Your body may be struggling to cope with energy production if you...

- Have energy slumps about an hour after eating
- Need to eat between meals to restore your energy
- Crave sugary or fatty foods
- Regularly use caffeine, alcohol or nicotine as an energy restorer

Your body may be poor at energy production if you...

- Have consistently low energy
- Your weight has gone up as your energy levels have gone down
- You always feel tired after eating a meal
- Stimulants and stimulation make you feel immediately exhausted

Creating The Right Mix

The two key components required to make energy are oxygen and glucose. A problem with energy production can therefore be the result of a shortage of either of these components, an imbalance between the two, or an inability to process them. You need molecules of both oxygen and glucose to make energy so if supplies or production of either is affected, then energy cannot be produced. We have already looked at how oxygen intake is reduced by excess or constant stress on the body. Too much short, shallow breathing brought on by stimulation or anxiety will give you an initial boost of energy but will reduce your oxygen intake over time, making your energy levels fall dramatically. In this situation, reduced oxygen intake is lowering energy production – however, if your body is stressed it will be demanding more energy. This means that energy levels are being reduced at a time when the body actually needs more. Low oxygen levels mean that you cannot utilize as much glucose to make energy, therefore it is irrelevant how much you have stored or put in because your body can only process it with the help of oxygen. So you can see that extremes or constant stress on the body can create a shortage of supply, imbalance existing supplies and upset the process of energy production. This is why it is so important to give your body regular breaks – because relaxation through deep breathing will restore oxygen levels, enabling your body to re-boost energy production. This means that your energy levels are more likely to remain stable throughout the day and your body will be more inclined to utilize your stored supplies to make energy, thus reducing the craving to snack on high-calorie quick fixes.

There are, of course, other factors that can decrease your oxygen intake. One of the most common is a polluted oxygen supply as a result of poor air quality in the environment or a self-induced source like smoking. One of the main reasons why people die from smoking is because nicotine destroys the tissue in the throat and lungs that is used to bring oxygen into the body. Without oxygen the body cannot make the energy it needs to operate so it ceases to function – it's as simple as that. Every cigarette smoked reduces your body's ability to produce energy, resulting in growing fatigue and potential health problems. Smoking is a perfect example of what I mean when I say that you are the only one that has ultimate control over your health. Health professionals like myself can present you with the facts but the choice is yours. If you want to have high energy levels and good health, then you have to face the fact that smoking won't give you either. Smoking may make you feel good for a short period, as well as having a calming effect on your nerves – which is why it is so hard to give up – but you have to accept that you will also feel tired and suffer from poor health in the long run. The fact is you cannot smoke and have good health – and the same may well apply to other lifestyle habits you have. Giving up damaging habits should not be thought of as depriving yourself of something, instead it should be seen as making a positive change that will help you achieve what you have always wanted – which is to feel good about yourself. If you are tired and run down, it may be that what you perceive as your only source of pleasure or stimulation is in fact your suppresser. Taking the healthy option will not deprive but liberate you to a happier, healthier life.

Keep Your Oxygen Intake Up

- If you're feeling tired, do some deep breathing.
- Take regular trips out into the countryside or walk in the park.
- Get friendly with plants – take up gardening.
- Don't smoke.
- Drink plenty of water, it is two-thirds oxygen.

Remember, you are always looking for balance so too much can be just as bad as too little. A healthy body will control how much oxygen it needs naturally, you just need to make sure you listen to what your body is telling you.

What's Fuelling You?

If you are suffering from health and fatigue problems generated by constant or extreme stress you may find that your body size and shape has changed. You may well have lost weight and muscle shape or piled on the pounds and feel you are swelling up. Dramatic weight loss can occur when the effects of constant stress or anxiety force adrenaline to shut down the digestive system for a prolonged period, making you disinterested in food. As fuel intake is reduced, this drop in resources forces the body to utilize every available supply of internal energy, starting with fat. Obviously this has some benefits for those with too much stored fat, but if your body is deprived of resources for too long and is forced to maintain high levels of stress and anxiety then it has to resort to converting muscle and body tissue into energy, resulting in muscle wasting, joint pains and fatigue. This exacerbates the situation as the body has less strength and power to cope with the on-going stress and anxiety and this can weaken it to a point were you could be forced to stop through weakness and fatigue.

For many of us, getting an adequate supply of fuel is never a problem because it comes from food and we love food. Any food containing starch, fat or sugar will supply the body with an energy source. One calorie is equal to one unit of energy so technically, the higher the calorie content, the greater the energy potential. And of course we're only too happy to eat all those energy-forming foods like chocolate, chips, biscuits and cakes because they happen to be our favourite types of food. There are two very good reasons why we like such foods so much: the first is because the higher the calorie, the greater the immediate energy rush and the second is that they also release happy drugs. We are supposed to enjoy food, otherwise we would have all died from starvation millions of years ago. A lot of today's health problems are due to the fact that these foods are so readily available – not because they are necessarily unhealthy. In addition, if you are unhappy and anxious with your life, you are more likely to crave these foods, as they become a rare source of pleasure and satisfaction.

We tend to look at calories as a bad thing but in theory the more calories you put in, the more energy you have to burn. Low-calorie diets do not work long term because they deprive the body of energy. It is very true that as a nation we are eating far too many calories but if you reduce your calorie intake too much you will also reduce your energy intake. If energy levels are low, then activity levels will be low, resulting in less calories burnt, hence another vicious cycle starts to emerge. In theory, if you cut down on calories, the body will utilize any excess stored energy to enable weight loss to occur without a drop in energy. So why do so many people today complain of being overweight and exhausted? Why isn't the theory working for them?

The problem is that your body becomes dependent on a consistent external supply because it can't or doesn't want to process its internal supply. This means that you will find it impossible to maintain a low-calorie diet because all your body wants you to do is continue eating. This, of course, makes you feel miserable and you turn to food not just as an energy source but as a mood enhancer.

We will look more closely at why your body finds it hard to process energy a little later but first let's look at how this might affect your weight. We have already seen how compulsive high-calorie foods are if you suffer from sudden slumps in energy or feel unhappy but here are some other classic reasons why you might suffer from low energy and weight gain.

1 CALORIE INTAKE IS TOO LOW: Too few calories and poor energy production will result in your body adopting a siege mentality. In the same way as there's a tendency to stockpile supplies when there is some sort of shortage but then refuse to use them for fear of running out, the body will not utilize stored energy supplies if it feels that there will be a limited supply for an indefinite period. This means it will store energy supplies rather than utilize them.
2 CRASH OR YO-YO DIETING: These are ineffective at maintaining a healthy weight because they upset the healthy metabolism of the body. One minute it is starved of food, the next minute it has too much. Over time this will put a great strain on the body's internal systems, exhausting the body further and causing emotional frustration and anxiety as motivational levels fall and lethargy sets in.
3 IRREGULAR EATING OR LIVING PATTERNS: If the body has no regular eating pattern or does not have a structure to follow then it cannot estimate how much energy it will need to deal with your demands, or when the next supply will be coming in. This forces it to hoard supplies and filter out only the bare minimum. When food comes along, your instinct will be to eat as much as possible because your body does not know how much energy it will need or when the next supply will turn up.
4 NOT EATING THE RIGHT CALORIES: As we have seen, the body needs quite a high daily calorie intake to supply it

with all the energy it needs. Some foods, such as those high in sugar and fat, give a fast release of energy, while others, such as potatoes and rice, release energy more slowly. Slow-release foods provide a more consistent supply of energy throughout the day, whereas fast-release foods will rush into the system and then quickly disappear. If your diet is high in fast-release foods then you will have slumps in energy soon after eating and will have to eat more often to keep energy levels up. These foods also overstress the system as you constantly jump from being over-stimulated to under-stimulated.

5 AN UNBALANCED DIET: To process energy, your body needs to utilize other essential nutrients, such as proteins, minerals and vitamins, to enable energy production to occur. If your diet is a typical western diet then it may well be high in energy-forming foods such as sugar, cereal and fat but low in the nutrients that are essential to enable your body to function. This means that the right energy components may be there but because of a lack of other elements, the body does not have the capability to convert them into usable energy, hence it stores them as fat.

If any of these scenarios relate to you then you need to concentrate on changing to a more balanced diet containing slow-energy-release foods, less stimulants and a greater mix of proteins, minerals and vitamins, and foods that that are free from additives and chemicals. Improvements to your health can also be made simply by following a regular eating pattern and putting more structure into your daily life, because if your body knows what it is doing it can calculate how many resources it needs to take in and this will reduce the desire to overeat. If your body knows when supplies will be replenished this will give it the security it needs to stop hoarding. If the body feels safe and in control then it is less inclined to over-stock and more inclined to produce available energy.

We often see excess weight as the problem when in fact it is more likely to be a symptom; the result of an imbalance generated by some sort of stress on the body. Having a healthy system will mean that you can eat well and have lots of energy, which will make you want to go out and be more active. You may well be sick of hearing the mantra 'eat less, exercise more', particularly if you have tried it and it didn't work. However, the key is your ability to generate energy, because if you get your system running effectively then unhealthy symptoms will begin to disappear of their own accord as energy levels start to rise.

Poor Energy Production

Now let's look at how your ability to produce energy declines as stress increases.

Your body needs a consistent supply of energy but this supply also needs to be flexible because sometimes you need to be able to generate that extra boost. Obviously your body has the ability to bring oxygen in on a continuous basis but with glucose (the body's primary source of fuel), the body needs a system of storage, otherwise you would have to eat continuously to keep energy production going. When you have eaten, a certain percentage of the food, i.e. the fast-energy-release foods such as sugar, will be converted into glucose and go straight into the bloodstream to meet up with oxygen molecules. This gives you your immediate supply of energy. The remainder of the food, which is a combination of the excess fast-release foods and the slow-release foods, such as rice, will be stored in your body cells. Only if there is a continual excess over time will it be stored as fat. For a healthy, active person this should not be a problem because they should be able to burn it off, as the body uses energy from its stored supplies in between meals. Body cells are like tea bags, they have a porous membrane that allows stored energy supplies to seep out into the bloodstream to meet up with oxygen and make energy. This enables you to have a continuous supply of energy. When supplies are running low, warning signs of hunger are generated to get you to top up your supplies. It is such a simple system and works very effectively, if you run your body the way it was designed to be run. However, if an imbalance occurs that affects this process, problems can soon begin. In order to take control of your own health, it is therefore vital that you understand how your body works best.

It's In The Cells

Virtually everything in the body is made from cells – your bones, muscles, tissues, organs and so on – and these cells are made predominantly from the nutrients you get from food. This means that you really are what you eat – you are basically just a composition of food components. These food components are not only the building blocks of your body but also enable your body to function – so to say a healthy diet is important to your health is a bit of an understatement. Each cell is an individual powerhouse with its own operational system, energy store and processing capacity. When we talk about wear and tear incurred by the body during stress or stimulation, it is the cells that bear the brunt of the damage. However, given adequate relaxation and essential resources, the body can repair this damage. Why is it then that some people's cells become so damaged that they are unable to process energy and to function effectively?

We have already looked at how a healthy system converts energy supplies into usable energy. The average body has around three trillion cells and when they fill up with energy supplies, they expand in size. And when three trillion cells expand in size, so do you. When you do something stimulating, you use up these supplies and, as the cells empty out, they decrease in size and so do you. This is how we balance our weight so that our body can store enough energy for emergencies without carrying excess fat – that is if the system is running effectively.

Oxidation

When your cellular structure is damaged as a result of an external force, such as a blow or a cut, or you experience the pain of an internal injury or invading bacteria, you are aware that your body is incurring some damage. However, the bulk of the wear and tear to your cells is a result of the natural process of burning energy. This is why your body needs an inbuilt repair and maintenance system, because it must have energy to survive but the production of energy takes its toll on the health and well-being of the body.

There are two key causes of on-going wear and tear to cells and both occur during stimulation. First, let's look at the effects of oxygen. Oxygen may seem like a pretty harmless substance but in fact it is one of the most explosive elements on the planet. I am sure everyone has done the experiment at school where you put a jar over a lighted candle and watch the flame go out. This happens because most fuel sources will only generate energy, in the form of heat, if oxygen is present – and producing bodily energy is no different. Glucose is our fuel source but we need oxygen to ignite it; it is quite literally your spark.

When a glucose and oxygen molecule meet up, they create an explosion that generates heat and power, just like an electric impulse. This is obviously an essential requirement because without that power source you wouldn't exist. Wear and tear occurs as a result of the explosive element of this process and the excessive heat it generates. You need to burn energy to live but that process involves small 'explosions' that cause damage to the cells. In addition, when energy burns, it generates heat and the higher the levels of stimulation the greater the heat. Excessive amounts of heat for too long will start to burn into the cells and create further damage. This process is known as oxidation, and it is a perfectly natural process that occurs when your body is stimulated. One of the purposes of relaxation is to deal with the effects of oxidation because during relaxation the body will cool down and cells will have an opportunity to repair themselves.

Oxidation only becomes a problem when the body is under extreme or prolonged stress, as this can cause cellular damage to become so great that it starts to affect the body's ability to function. Remember, virtually everything in the body is made from cells and this is why symptoms of stress are so diverse and wide-ranging – because oxidation can affect cellular structure anywhere in the body. The process of cell recovery is not only dependent on the relaxation process, it also requires the right components to repair and replace cells. These components are found in certain foods, such as vegetables. This is why such foods are referred to as antioxidants, because they contain the nutrients required by the body to repair the cellular damaged generated when you stimulate your body into action.

There are two top tips to beat the effects of oxidation:

1. Give you body time to relax.
2. Eat a healthy, balanced diet.

Free Those Radicals

An additional, potentially damaging effect of oxidation comes in the form of free radicals. These are unstable molecules that are created in the normal process of oxidation. These unstable molecules contain an unpaired electron (electrons are normally joined in pairs) which, in an attempt to become stable, will try to break into another molecule and steal one of its electrons. If it succeeds it destabilizes that molecule, which now becomes a free radical and goes off to break up some more cellular structure.

Confused? Well think of it this way – electrons need to be in a pair so an unpaired electron will attempt to nick an electron from a healthy cell, damaging it in the process. This creates a domino effect as free radicals create more free radicals. Obviously it pays to nip this process in the bud – and the body is capable of doing this as part of its regular maintenance and repair programme. Problems occur when your natural healing process is prevented from operating effectively due to lack of resources and poor maintenance (i.e. a lack of antioxidant foods in the diet), excesses and extremes of prolonged stress and anxiety, or as a result of overloading the system with irritants such as alcohol, caffeine and chemicals that cause free radicals.

If I wanted to be ill, tired, fat and miserable again, I could probably achieve that in a couple of weeks by going back to my old diet, my high stimulant intake, my overstressed attitude to life and my disregard for my health but it now involves hardly any effort at all for me to run my system effectively because I benefit so greatly from the results. I didn't mean to cause harm, I didn't even realize that I was – and I accept that I am now not 'miss healthy angel' who will never be ill again – but I do now know that I am the one with ultimate control over my health and well-being. My environment may conspire against my body but I am certainly not going to add to that.

The Truth About Toxins

The second key area of natural damage generated by energy production is a result of the build up of toxic waste. If you look at fuel sources such as petrol or coal for example, during the burning process a residue is produced. This needs to be cleared away once the energy has been utilized, in order to enable a new supply to burn effectively. This clear-up operation is necessary for two main reasons: the first is because it clogs everything up, preventing oxygen reaching the fuel source; and the second is that it is toxic and contains harmful by-products that could be dangerous. Our internal energy supply is no different. As we utilize energy, a residue or by-product is produced and this needs to be disposed of, otherwise it will get in the way and cause damage.

Your structure is made up of bones, muscles and tissue, each of which is a mass of cells stacked together to create form. In between the individual cells, fluid flows, supplying the essential nutrients and water the cells need to function. This fluid also transports oxygen around the body so that it can fuse with the glucose oozing out of the cells and supply energy to all areas of the body. Cells themselves are an individual powerhouse so in order to function they also need energy. This means that your body needs energy to make energy. To maintain energy levels and keep the cells healthy it is essential that nothing affects this constant flow. In addition to supplying energy, this distribution system also removes harmful substances, enables a speedy response to any damage that is incurred and allows the immune system to operate effectively.

When your body burns energy, the process leaves behind a residue. This residue needs to be disposed of quickly because it contains acids that are toxic to the body, hence the name toxin. If the toxins are not removed this acid will burn into the cellular structure, causing damage. Again, it is a naturally occurring process and yes, you guessed it, toxins are disposed of by the body during relaxation. I think you can start to see a pattern emerging when I say that toxins only become a problem when your body is exposed to extreme or prolonged periods of stress or anxiety, it lacks the essential resources required to combat them or there is a high intake of stimulating substances or chemicals that overload your system with toxins.

Toxins weaken your cellular strength through acidity, making it harder for your body to function effectively – but they also have a dramatic effect on energy levels if they are allowed to build up.

This is because they create a deposit. In the same way as burnt wood makes ash and gas generates soot, toxins form crystals that build up in your system. As they grow into a bigger mass they start to block and clog up the freeflowing system in the body, preventing effective waste disposal and the distribution of nutrients and energy.

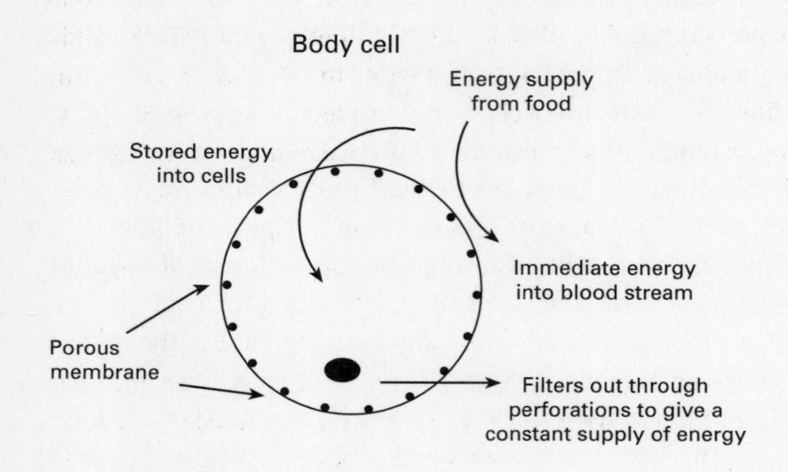

Effects of the decline in health of a cell from oxidation, free radicals and toxins

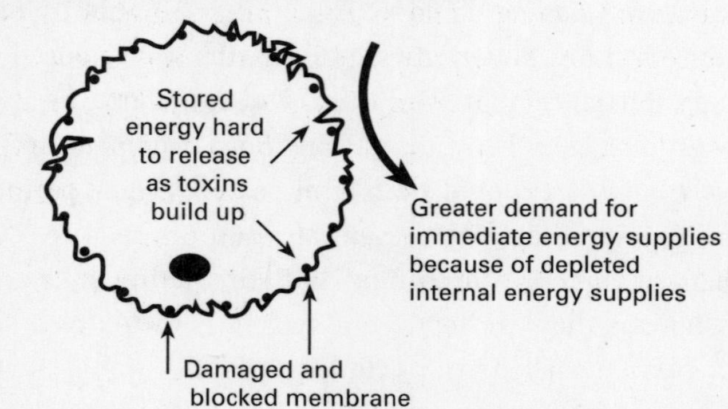

A Burning Example

Think about the hob on a gas cooker. It has a ring of tiny holes around it that lets the gas seep out into the oxygen-rich atmosphere, thus allowing the gas to burn. The process of cooking results in spills that make a mess around the burner and a sooty residue that is produced by the burning gas. If the hob is cleaned regularly then the mess is easy to clean away but, if it is left to build up, it becomes ingrained onto the hob, making it harder to clear up. If this mess is allowed to continue building up it could start to block up the holes in the burner, preventing the flow of gas. If this occurs, it is irrelevant how much gas you have stored away, if it cannot get into the atmosphere, no heat and therefore no energy will be produced. As more and more holes are clogged up with waste and residue, less and less energy can be utilized, making it virtually impossible for you to cook effectively.

Now think about how your cells store and distribute energy. It is very similar to a gas hob. You need to have a continuous but variable supply of energy. Your body has a supply of stored fuel that needs oxygen to utilize that energy. These supplies are filtered out through holes in the cell wall to supply your body with the energy it needs. This process uses up resources, creates waste and damage, and makes a mess – and all these consequences need to be continuously addressed in order to keep the process of energy production running smoothly and your body in full working order. Your body does all the production work; your job is to make sure production is maintained by providing a consistent supply of high-quality fuel and the right conditions for the process to work as it should.

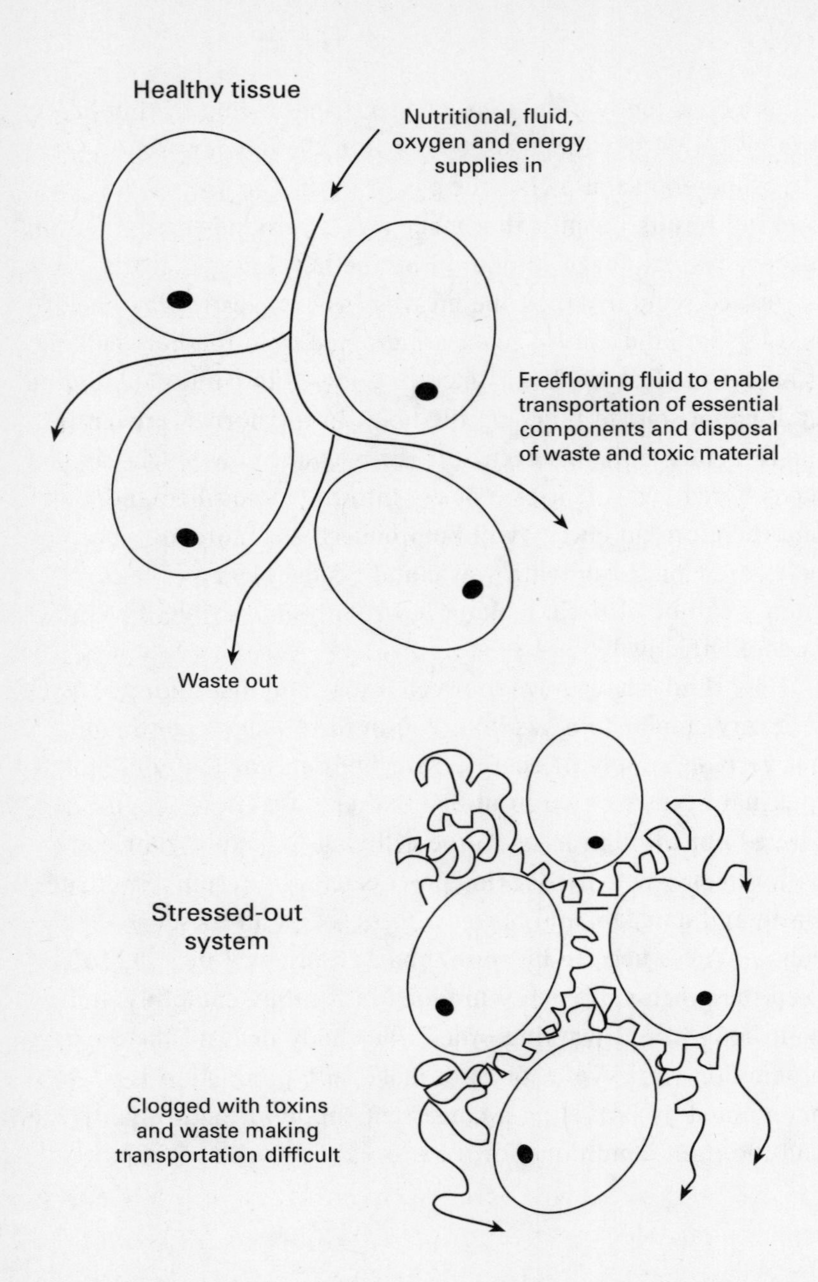
Healthy tissue
Nutritional, fluid, oxygen and energy supplies in
Freeflowing fluid to enable transportation of essential components and disposal of waste and toxic material
Waste out
Stressed-out system
Clogged with toxins and waste making transportation difficult

An Example

Let's imagine that you eat something and, just as an example, your body uses 25 per cent of the usable glucose in that food source as an initial energy source. It goes straight into the bloodstream to be fused with oxygen as an instant source of energy. Therefore you have 75 per cent left to be stored away in your body cells. Now in a healthy system, once this supply had been processed, the energy would be available and the body would want to use it. You would therefore feel energized and restless to be active. That is the healthy response; but what if your body had trouble processing that energy because of the wear and tear of constant stress, a lack of resources or an overload of toxins?

This would make you feel exhausted because your body would be having trouble utilizing the stored energy and would have to rely more heavily on the smaller amount of immediate energy that is available after eating. This would mean that your body would not be able to maintain a continuous supply of energy so your energy levels would fluctuate dramatically throughout the day, depending on when and what you ate. You would only get an energy boost when you ate, making you more inclined to snack and increase your food intake. If this continually occurs then your body will start to become dependent on getting its energy from this small and short-lived immediate supply but you would still be storing a large percentage of the unprocessed energy in your cells, causing your weight to rise. In this example, your body is only getting 25 per cent of the potential energy available to it so your energy levels will be low, making your body panic in desperation to boost those levels. In this dysfunctional situation the only immediate options available are to either eat foods that are higher in immediate energy or turn to stimulants that shock the body into stimulation. If this is the case, you will start to crave foods that are high in sugar and fat – like chocolate, biscuits and cheese –

or increase your intake of alcohol, salt, nicotine or caffeine. An imbalance in the body has created these cravings but the fact that your body has become reliant on these 'stimulants' means that your consumption of them could increase to a consistently high level. This then generates more work for your body and increases the wear and tear on it, pushing it even further out of balance, which results in further fatigue and potential health and well-being problems.

Toxic Alert

How toxic are you? You will be adding toxins to your system if you...

- Drink alcohol
- Smoke
- Drink fizzy drinks, especially if they contain sweeteners or caffeine
- Sleep badly
- Don't exercise
- Over-exercise
- Eat processed food
- Use chemically-based toiletries
- Live in a city

Your body is designed to deal with toxins because it makes plenty of its own, so if your body is running effectively you can cope with and enjoy, for example, a glass of wine, a cup of coffee or an apartment in central London. However, if your system is worn out and ineffective it needs all the help it can get to recover. The more unbalanced your system becomes, the more sensitive it becomes to anything that adds to the toxic overload, hence it will start to react negatively to things it was once happy to tolerate. Unfortunately, these are usually the things we class as pleasurable and we are therefore reluctant to give them up – but there is no benefit in indulgence if the effects are fatigue and poor health.

Looking After Your Cells

The symptoms of stress and anxiety, whether physical or mental, can affect any system of the body due to the damage they cause at a cellular level. Cells have a life span so they are always in the process of being renewed. That means that by the end of the year you will probably have a completely different set of cells from those you had only a year earlier – so theoretically that means a new you. When a cell needs to be replaced, it clones itself so that the replacement cell can continue doing the same job without any disruption to the body. If you have healthy cells, then these will be replaced by healthy cells but, if your cells have suffered from damage and are weakened by lack of resources, you will end up with weak cells that could become damaged or dysfunctional. This means that your cells will be less able to cope with the things you throw at it, and a continuing lack of resources will weaken it still further. When these cells are replaced, they are more likely to be badly put together and less likely to function effectively. This makes your body even less able to cope and so it goes on. If we put this into context, your cells make you, the person, so if you have had a particularly difficult year, continuously poor diet or just been burning the candle at both ends for too long then, by the end of the year, your health and well-being will go into decline. This is why health problems emerge over time rather than just appearing – it is the result of your body slowly crumbling under the pressure.

The good news is that you can improve the condition of your cells pretty quickly. The more you invest in the early stages, the quicker the results. As I have already explained, your body does its own repairing, you just need to create the right environment to enable that to happen. It will have taken more than one thing over time to finally tip the balance of your health, so the best way to recovery is to use a strategy that combines everything that benefits your body and excludes anything that doesn't.

The Combination Recovery Plan

- Run your stress response right.
- Get plenty of positive stimulation.
- Incorporate relaxation.
- Put the right resources in.
- Keep potentially harmful substances out.

These are the five points you need to concentrate on to achieve good health. We have already covered some of these points but as you read on you will start to see why it is so important to consider them all. I have made some initial suggestions as to how you can begin to achieve successful results but you, as an individual, need to find out which ones are particularly relevant to you. However, you should think of it as a war on five fronts because without tackling each problem area to some extent, your overall success will be limited.

Health Conditions

Because all body tissue is made of cells, the negative effects they undergo from an unhealthy imbalance can be found anywhere in the body. Here we look at some typical stress-related health problems but there are many more that are generated or influenced by upsetting the healthy balance of your body.

SKIN: The skin is usually first to be affected by an imbalance, as it is the body's extremity. Supplies of energy and nutrients have the furthest to travel in order to reach the skin, so it is more likely to be affected by blockages and lack of power in the body's transportation system. Also, the skin has more continuous exposure to the outside world than any other system in the body so it gets a constant battering, making it harder to maintain healthy cells. The combination of these factors, and the fact that skin cells are constantly having to be renewed, means that skin problems are at the forefront of stress-related illness.

The first signs are poor skin quality, dullness in colour and black rings under the eyes. Over time, other problems emerge, such as dry and flaky skin, adult acne and cysts or red blotches or rashes. Stress skin conditions include cold sores, mouth ulcers, eczema, dermatitis and chilblains.

MUSCLES: Your muscles use a huge amount of energy so their cellular structure is particularly affected by prolonged and excessive use. Remember, it is not just the muscles you consciously control that are affected by power loss and wear and tear, it is also those internal muscles that power things like your digestive system. Lactic acid is the main toxin that builds up in the muscles and as crystals form and acids build up, your muscle cells will start to tire and burn up. This produces weak and sensitive muscles that are sore to touch. Not only does this make you feel physically weak but consider the effect on those unconscious internal muscles – they will also start to slow down and become dysfunctional, affecting their capability.

BONE: When your body is constantly under stress it becomes very acidic. One of the ways your body deals with acidity is to use calcium to neutralize it. Your kidneys utilize calcium to deal with these acids, as it condenses them into urine. However, the body must obtain this calcium from somewhere and if there isn't enough in your diet, or there are high levels of acid in your system, the body will start to use the calcium in your bones. This means that your bones are being broken down to deal with a problem elsewhere in the body. Your bones are a cellular structure, like everything else, so they will still be affected by the usual cellular damage incurred from stress or poor diet but at the same time they are also being stripped of resources to deal with those problems. It's hardly surprising then that skeletal problems can be a feature of an imbalanced system.

GLANDS AND HORMONES: Dotted around inside the head and body are numerous glands that control the body's coping mechanisms. By releasing hormones, they regulate numerous essential but diverse processes in the body, such as sleep, blood sugar, stress, sexual urges and immune responses. They are all made from cells and all supply on demand. The thyroid, for example, controls your metabolism. If your metabolic rate needs to rise because your body needs additional stimulation, then it will produce more thyroxine, the hormone that controls your metabolism, to give you the boost you need. This is a normal, healthy reaction. However, if your body is exposed to constant or extreme amounts of stress it will find it hard to keep up with the continual demand that results from having to keep your metabolism running on high, and it will begin to tire. As it is a cellular structure, it is also affected by the wear and tear caused by this continuous high stimulation, because it is being asked to increase production but is capable of less.

The problem of high demand but low capability is a common one throughout the body, and glands and their ability to regulate your body with hormonal production are no different. The adrenal glands that release the hormones required to trigger the stress response, such as adrenaline and cortisol, can also burn out under extreme or prolonged pressure, as will the pancreas. The pancreas regulates blood sugar with the help of insulin. We have already seen how energy production affects the balance of glucose in our body and, if an imbalance occurs, the pancreas will be forced to work overtime. If this is maintained, it will start to tire and be unable to keep up the high levels of insulin production required, throwing your blood sugar levels all over the place. This results in massive energy fluctuations and, in the most serious cases, diabetes. Incidentally, the pancreas also supplies the gut with digestive juices, so a poorly performing pancreas can cause problems for other body systems. This is why you cannot isolate health problems – a problem anywhere in the body can have a knock-on effect over the whole body.

Immune To Everything

Your body has to work hard every day. For example, your kidneys filter 425 gallons of blood a day, while your liver has to perform more than 500 different functions. The heart, blood, lungs, sexual organs ... everything operates within a cellular structure that is constantly bombarded with abuse.

Dealing with everyday functions and the wear and tear they generate is the responsibility of the body's inbuilt repair and maintenance programme. However, the body also has to cope with exposure to potentially harmful substances and dangerous situations on a daily basis and for this it requires an immune system. The immune system is also a cellular system and reduced immune responses make the body more vulnerable to disease and illness and less capable of repairing injury. However, the stress response can mask signs that we are ill or that our immune system is not functioning as it should. The stress response has the ability to reduce pain and inflammation through the action of cortisol (this is another reason why positive stimulation makes us feel good). When the stress response is activated, the aim is to achieve a quick and effective result and because pain and inflammation would be a hindrance, it holds them off. It is often not until the body relaxes, that the full extent of the damage incurred during stimulation is experienced. I am sure you have experienced those feeling of complete exhaustion that only appear after you have finished something stressful or stimulating. Such symptoms are a sign that the body is suffering and unfortunately such signals can only be suppressed for so long.

An Example Of Overload

I am sure that you have a cupboard or drawer where you put your 'not sure what to do with or no time to deal with but must sort out one day' stuff. Over time, the drawer or cupboard fills up as you delay dealing with any of it and continue to try and jam stuff in. One day you put in one thing too many and the bottom collapses or the doors won't close and you are then forced to sort out the mess. Imagine the same process happening in your body. Take your immune system for example – every day it is bombarded with jobs to do, some important, some it can come back to. If it is constantly overloaded, the workload will start to build up but its ability to deal with it all is reducing, therefore more and more things are being put to one side to be dealt with later. Eventually it gets to a point where these jobs cannot be put off any longer and your problems become overwhelming. You are then forced to stop completely and spend a few days in bed while your immune system tries to get things straight again. These are the days where you feel ill but you are not suffering from anything specific, you just feel worn out or 'a bit fluey'.

The body is more vulnerable to colds and infection when it is physically run down. This is an important factor in whether or not you catch or develop whatever bug is going around – otherwise an epidemic would affect everyone. When you are run down, your immune system is less capable of dealing with the challenges that are constantly presented to it. Our environment is full of potentially harmful bacteria and particles but when our health is good we are hardly ever aware of them because we have a strong immune system. It is only when the system breaks down that these external negative elements can really start to have a detrimental effect on our health.

The Jug of Ill Health

This is how your body maintains a healthy internal balance

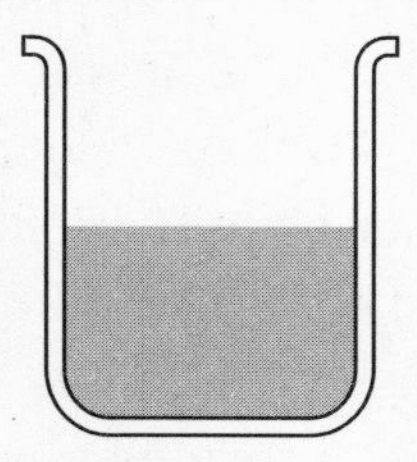

The stress and stimulation of living builds up a backlog of problems for your body to deal with...

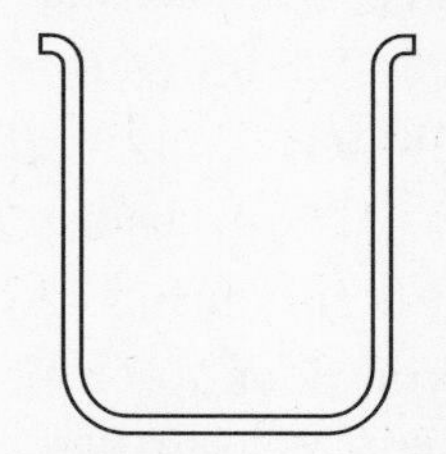

...but when you rest and relax, your body then deals with these problems, restoring the balance.

This is how that balance is lost

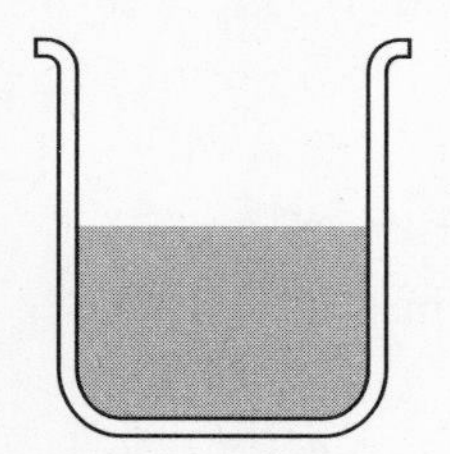

If these problems are not dealt with, then the backlog remains. At this stage, small niggly ailments and a drop in stamina appear.

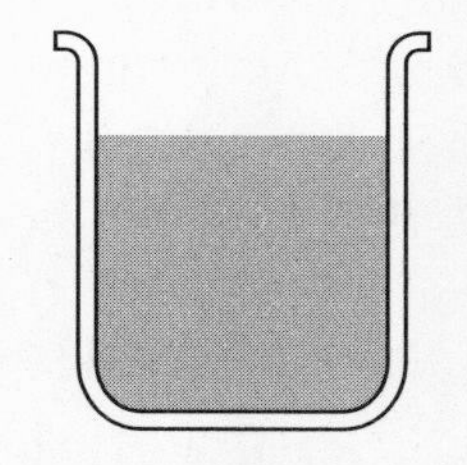

If this situation continues, then the backlog increases in size and builds up as existing problems create new problems. At this stage conditions and fatigue are likely to become chronic.

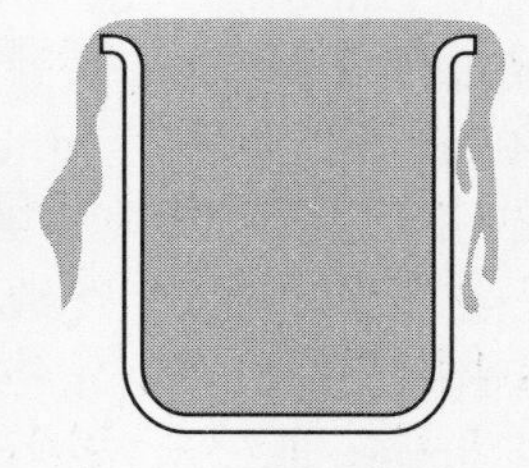

Finally a bout of illness or ill health will force you to stop and rest as your body will be overflowing with problems and no longer able to cope with the stress.

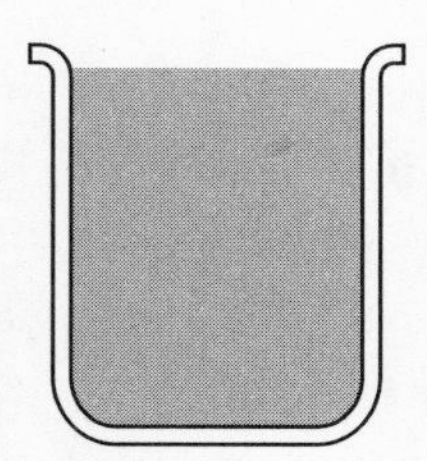

This rest will stop the overflow and enable you to get going again, but with reduced ability.

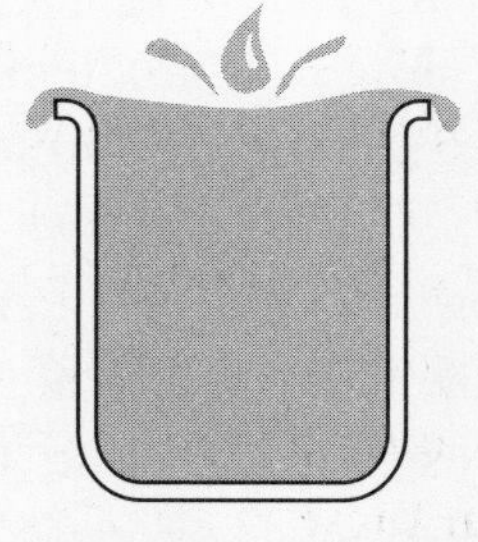

But it only takes one small drop of stress to push your system over the edge again if your body is deprived of the additional care it needs at this stage to restore the balance back to a healthy level.

Prevent The Backlog Building Up

It is perfectly natural that in the process of using your body you will generate maintenance jobs for it to do. This could be cell repair or renewal, toxin disposal or processing new resources. These jobs have to be stacked up until your body has time to deal with them during rest, therefore to maintain a healthy balance you have to ensure that these jobs never get too big or that your body has the time and resources to sort them out before new jobs appear. If this doesn't happen, a backlog will start to build up. Now imagine that you have a big jug inside your body that contains this backlog – just as your drawer or cupboard contains your outstanding paperwork. This storage space allows your body to deal with the continuing ongoing or immediate tasks at hand without disruption. If the amount of work builds up due to lack of time and resources then your jug will start to fill. Initially, this shouldn't be a problem because there will be plenty of room in the jug. Over time you may experience a few niggling little health problems and a drop in stamina as it starts to fill – although they are problems that can be easily suppressed with a potion, lotion or energy-boosting stimulant. However, these symptoms are early warning signs and if the cause of them is not addressed and the overload continues, the jug will keep on filling up. Originally these small, unnecessary jobs were not a priority but, the longer they are left, the more of a problem they become.

As the amount of unresolved jobs and their urgency grows, so does the speed at which your jug fills up because your body is finding it harder to function effectively. Health problems could now become chronic and more severe but remain either undiagnosed or incurable. In this case, all your doctor can do is give you stronger drugs to deal with the symptoms. This means that you can still function but it also means that the cause is left unresolved and the jug continues to fill. Finally your jug will become so full that it will start to overflow. This is the point when the body forces you to stop, as it cannot continue. Unfortunately you will think that whatever it was that pushed you over the edge – be it an illness, emotional trauma or accident – is the reason for your poor state of health when in fact the initial problem could have started well before that as a result of a multitude of small but growing stresses over a period of time. As I have said many times before, a healthy body is designed to deal with trauma and illness, but a weakened one cannot.

Once you have had time to rest, a degree of recovery will occur but if no effort is made to empty the jug then it will only take one small problem to push you back over the edge into chronic ill health and fatigue. When I was ill, any slight improvement made me want to go out and take over the world – but, of course, acting on this urge always resulted in an immediate decline. So take it from me, if you don't give your body an opportunity to clear up the backlog and give it the resources to do so, then your jug will always be overflowing. If you want to say yes to good health then the first thing you need to do is look at the demands, requirements and well-being of your body because when your body says no, what it's really saying is 'I need help'.

How To Increase Your Energy

1 TAKE A COMBINATION OF POSITIVE STEPS

It is very rarely one big thing that upsets your health and well-being but more a combination of negative aspects that build up over time, making your body less resilient to the stresses and strains of living. When the body is bogged down with a multitude of small but on-going imbalances it will find it harder to cope with a sudden emergency or trauma or have no energy left over to have fun. The route to energy recovery involves addressing the negative aspects that have lead to, or are maintaining, a strain on the body, and introducing a combination of positive steps that will improve your health. Remember the Five Points to Recovery (see page 58). In part three these are the starting points to recovery so keep them in mind as you continue reading.

2 DON'T CLOG YOUR SYSTEM UP WITH UNNECESSARY TOXINS

Your body produces plenty of toxins of its own so if you want to run your body at a high level of stimulation, you need to keep it as clear as possible. Anything chemical, complex or processed and anything that over-stimulates or upsets the body will generate more toxins. If you want lots of energy, don't push your system into overload or irritate it with small but persistent abuses without giving it a break.

3 GIVE YOUR BODY TIME TO CLEAR UP THE MESS

Any sort of stimulation, whether it is positive or negative, will use up resources and generate wear and tear, so you need to give your body time to rest and restore. Exercise, for example, is a useful stress-relieving tool and a good way of keeping healthy but it is something that instigates the stress response and therefore has the ability to drain resources and generate damage from oxidation and toxic build up. The reason your body builds up muscle and stamina through physical activity is due to your demand – it's a case of 'use it or lose it'. Too little activity causes wasting because if you don't express a demand, the body sees no reason why it should put effort into maintaining muscle you appear not to need. When you exercise regularly you are asking your body to do an action again and again. If your body initially finds it cannot fulfil your demand because it does not have enough energy or strength, it will concentrate on improvements. Your body will build new cells to hold more energy and add strength to muscles to achieve an easy and successful result. However, it can only do that building work while you are in a state of rest and relaxation – therefore, if you want to be fit, you also need to relax.

4 FEED YOUR BODY WELL
We have already looked at the importance of putting the right resources in your body and keeping harmful substances out and in the next section we shall look more closely at diet. Your body needs a balanced and varied diet to maintain good health, so if you want to keep your energy levels up, you need to eat for energy.

5 MAINTAIN YOUR ENERGY LEVELS
Take small steps throughout the day to keep your energy high, rather than waiting for it to fall before you address it – it's a lot easier. Remember to do your micro relaxation breaks (see page 36), keep topping up your fluid levels and eat regular meals. Look out for those early warning signs and ask yourself why you are starting to feel tired. Is it because you have not had a break for ages, not had breakfast or not had a drink perhaps? Don't wait until your body has run out of energy because you will be more inclined to reach for those damaging short-term, quick-fix solutions. Aim for long-term energy maintenance by keeping up with your body's demands.

Nourishment For Life

What you put into your body has a huge effect on what you get out of it. Yes your body needs food and water to function – but it can't be just any old food or fluid. Your body has thousands of different components and a vast array of tasks to carry out and in order to do everything demanded of it, it requires a large number of nutrients. The choice is simple, you either put things in that give you energy, enable your body to function and deal with cell repair and maintenance so that you look and feel good, or you don't. We have already looked at the importance of food as an energy source but it also provides the building blocks of life, your life in fact. Your cellular structure is built and maintained predominately from the elements you obtain from food and your essential body functions are run by these nutrients. If health professionals like myself always seem to be droning on about eating a healthy, balanced and varied diet, it is simply because we are trying to keep you alive and well.

- Your body needs a varied diet because...
  Providing your body with its essential nutritional requirements is just like building a jigsaw puzzle each day. There are loads of different pieces that all interlock to make a complete picture. If there is just one bit missing then the picture will remain unfinished. Just like a collector needs to have one of each to make a set of any value, so your body needs to have a full set of nutrients and the right type of fluid.
- Your body needs a balanced diet because...
  No one food item contains all the nutrients and fluids you need so there is no point eating lots of one type of nutrient and neglecting the others. The body will be unable to use any oversupply and will have to go to the trouble of finding somewhere to store it or dispose of it unused, thus creating storage and waste removal problems. By repeatedly eating the same foods over and over again, you will be depriving your body of the other nutrients that are essential to make everything work together. Nutrients and fluids rarely work independently, they usually need other elements to enable them to do their job, which is why it is so important to have a balanced diet.

Too Much Or Too Little For Too Long

The phrase 'everything in moderation' may be one you are only too familiar – and bored – with, but, as we have already established, the body only has one pet hate and that is extremes of things for too long. Forget about classifying foods as inherently good or bad, think in terms of too much or too little for too long as the main route to nutritional malnourishment. I have had many clients who insist that they have an extremely healthy diet and changing it will only make matters worse. However, if you are having health problems it is important to re-examine your diet – regardless of whether or not you think it is healthy.

Case History

I had one very frustrated client who suffered from anxiety, fatigue and adult acne. She was adamant that she could not shift the few pounds she had wanted to lose, despite changing her diet and activity regime to one that she felt could not be made any healthier. Every day, for some years, she had been going to the gym for three hours and eating only fruit for breakfast and lunch and an undressed salad for dinner. Not only was this lifestyle unhealthy for her physically, it provided very little in the way of pleasure or satisfaction. She experienced no reward as a result of all her hard labour and it took up so much of her time that she had none left to go out and enjoy life. Her body was undernourished and over-stimulated and she was emotionally unhappy because of her self-imposed regime. The easiest way of knowing if your lifestyle is a healthy one is to listen to your body. If you feel happy and healthy then you must be doing something right. She was unhappy with her life and was still unhealthy so it would appear that her health regime wasn't working. It was not surprising to me that her body was in a poor state but she took some convincing. It's not every day you are told to eat and relax more if you want to feel and look better.

Eating For Balance

The problem with taking health advice in isolation is that it gives you a good verses bad image of health management. If you class something as good then, theoretically, the more you do of it, the healthier you become. Conversely, it means that anything that is bad needs to be avoided at all costs. Thankfully, the body does not operate like that. Think back to how your stress response works: it is vital, enjoyable and satisfying to implement but it still has a down side. Similarly, not using your stress response enough also has a down side. The same sort of process applies to what you put into your body and a similar balancing act is required.

There are always payoffs to be made, no matter how healthy or unhealthy things are perceived to be. For example, fruit is full of vitamins but is also high in sugar and acid, prawns are low in fat and full of protein but very high in cholesterol, and milk is a good source of calcium but also has a complex make-up that can make digestion difficult. This is why balance is so important. It is also vital to consider your own individual needs. If you are lactose-intolerant or allergic to seafood then milk or prawns are not a healthy option for you, while those with a blood sugar problem could benefit from restricting their intake of fruits that are particularly high in sugar. Following a diet that is appropriate to you is crucially important in finding your own level of health and well-being – even if it doesn't appear to tally with the general advice.

The Basic Requirements

Basically you need carbohydrates and fats for energy (although under stress your body can convert protein into energy), proteins and essential fatty acids for cell growth and repair, vitamins to run body functions and minerals to do a bit of both.

CARBOHYDRATES ARE FOUND IN: Fruit, vegetables, cereals, sugar, honey and milk.
FATS ARE FOUND IN: Butter, margarine, oils, nuts, cheese, milk, meat and oily fish such as salmon.
PROTEINS ARE FOUND IN: Meat, fish, seafood, nuts, eggs, seeds and pulses.
MINERALS AND VITAMINS ARE FOUND IN: There are numerous sources but the highest concentration is found in meat, fish, vegetables, fruit, nuts, seeds, milk and pulses.

These lists indicate the main component but many of these foods contain a combination of the essential nutrients required by your body but all in different quantities and ratios.

- If you eat lots of dairy produce, potatoes, bread, cereal and pasta, and not much meat, fish, green vegetables and nuts then your diet is high in energy-forming foods and low in repair and maintenance foods. If your diet consists mainly of carbohydrate or fat-based foods then you will have lots of energy supplies going in but there may not be a wide enough range of nutrients to enable your body to process those energy supplies. This could cause digestive processes to slow down and clog up, resulting in fatigue, weight gain and cellular health problems such as poor skin quality. On the other hand, if your diet is too low in these energy foods, you will have no obvious energy supply so the body will have to use protein as a source of energy. This means that there will be less protein available for repair and maintenance but more tissue wasting because the protein in muscles, for example, will be stripped out. This could lead to physical weakness, reduced immunity and fatigue.
- If you eat lots of cakes, biscuits, chocolate and processed foods and drink lots of coffee, fizzy drinks and alcohol and you have little in the way of vegetables, meat, fish, potatoes, nuts, seeds and pulses, then your diet is low in essential

nutrients and high in fast-energy-release foods and stress-inducing stimulants. These create immediate energy rushes followed by energy crashes. A diet like this will generate high levels of stress on your body and cause a build up of excessive amounts of toxins and cell damage if sustained for too long. This can result in dramatic drops in energy, weight fluctuations and excess acid problems, such as abdominal pain and cystitis.

To say that changing my diet made a difference to my health is an understatement. At the time I had no comprehension of the importance of diet. Of course I knew I needed food for energy and that without it I would die, but I never really grasped the concept that diet was a big factor in the state of my health. Over the years since then it has become obvious to me that there are a great many people who vastly underestimate just how interlinked diet and health are. I was amazed when a client said to me, 'I have had IBS for over ten years and you are the first person who has ever suggested that it could be related to my diet.'

It may seem obvious to me now that there has to be a link between a problem with your digestive system and what you put into it but, when I was ill, I probably would not have made the connection either because the advice available tended to focus on finding an alien physical irritant or a psychosomatic cause. During my illness I saw a dietician who told me that my diet was fine but, even if it wasn't, it would make very little difference to my state of health. Nowadays I can see that my diet then was appallingly unhealthy but, scarily, so typical in western society today.

Digestive Dilemmas

Apart from the commonplace problem of poor health through poor diet, there are two other main reasons why the food we eat can adversely affect our health. The first is as a result of genetics or an inherent problem that has produced a weakness or irregularity in the body; the second is a decline in the health of the digestive system due to illness, injury or stress. Genetic or inherent problems can usually only be controlled and not cured and require the sufferer to take additional care to keep the condition under control. For example, a diabetes sufferer has to take extra special care with their diet and an allergy sufferer has to avoid the foods they react to if they want to stay healthy. If you are already aware of a weak spot in your system then it is doubly important that you take good care of your overall health – this also applies to those who do not have a readily identifiable problem but are aware that they have a sensitive system.

Many general digestive problems are a result of food sensitivities, bacteria build up or acid overload from negative aspects of lifestyle, such as stress and poor diet. The problem with this is that the symptoms are often vague and produce nothing diagnosable. They can also be attributed to a general decline in health due to stress and poor diet because this is how they were initially sparked off.

Could Your Problem Be Caused By Food?

Do you suffer from excessive abdominal bloating?
Do you have chronic symptoms?
Do you suffer from an 'unspecified' illness such as ME or IBS?
Do you have problems with your bowel movements?
Do you suffer from bladder discomfort?
Do you suffer from thrush?
Do you suffer from abdominal or lower back pain?
Do you suffer from constant headaches?
Do you suffer from skin problems?
Do you suffer from constant fatigue?
Do you suffer from burning sensations or acid problems in your stomach?

If you regularly experience problems with such symptoms, then it could be a result of what you eat. To understand why, you first need to look at the relationship between the digestive system and the rest of the body because they are, of course, closely linked. A dysfunctional digestive system can cause a vicious circle of problems. A weak system will find it hard to process food, so you develop a sensitivity to those foods that are hardest to digest, such as wheat and dairy produce. However, because you can often pinpoint the fact that these foods are causing a problem, they often become the main focus for your attention. Having excluded them from your diet, you may well experience some degree of recovery but your digestive system is still being put under strain because the original reason for the weakness has not been addressed. This increases the chance of you developing more sensitivities, not just to food but to other substances in your environment, which pushes you further into poor health and a restrictive diet and lifestyle. Therefore to deal with food sensitivities you need to be concerned with the health of your whole body and not simply what you put into it.

Digestive Decline

The digestive system is likely to be the first system to be affected by stress and a poor diet but often without any immediate direct symptoms. This is because the digestive symptom has to manufacture resources for the whole of the body, so often negative symptoms emerge elsewhere as supplies of energy and nutrients begin to dry up.

The digestive system, like everything else in the body, is a cellular structure. It breaks down food, extracting what it needs at various stages in the process and disposes of what it doesn't need, along with the usual collection of toxic wastes generated during metabolism. As with everything in the body, the digestive system needs energy to power it, nutrients to repair and maintain it and a balance of stimulation and relaxation to keep it running effectively. The digestive system is a multi-tasker; it is designed to deal with a variety of demands, stresses and strains, toxic chemicals, bacteria and an irregular flow of substances. It can therefore put up with a lot but, like everything else in the body, it cannot tolerate extremes of anything for too long. This could be too much of the same foods, too much food, too little food, not enough nutrients, too many chemicals, too much processed or complex food, too many stimulants, too much waste, not enough fluid, too much bacteria, too much acid or too much stress.

Food Sensitivity

The problem of 'extremes' relates back to my earlier point about food sensitivities. Many people consider themselves sensitive to wheat and milk – they have given them up and feel much better, therefore they decide they must have some sort of inherent intolerance to them. In fact, for most people, it is more likely they have simply been eating too much for too long and overloading their system.

Western diets rely heavily on these two food sources and research shows that we are overeating them at the expense of other foods. For example, if your daily diet consisted of a cereal for breakfast, a sandwich for lunch and pasta for dinner, you might consider it quite varied but the body would see it as wheat, wheat and more wheat. Wheat is a fibrous and complex food source and it is these two factors that make it beneficial – in moderation. It takes a long time to digest, it releases its energy slowly and it contains lots of fibre, which helps with the disposal of toxic waste, but all of these factors also mean that it involves a good deal more effort to process than other basic food sources and it also produces more waste. For an overloaded system, this is very stressful so it becomes sensitive to it.

For example, if you eat wheat at every meal this can, over time, create a backlog of ineffectively processed wheat in the gut, clogging your system up and tiring it out. This inability to process and dispose of waste will then have a knock-on effect on the rest of the body as toxins build up and nutritional supplies to the body are reduced. This can then create cellular damage and weakening in all the body's systems. Let's not forget that your digestive system is tied in with the other systems and processes of the body. For example, it needs the heart to pump energy to it, the brain to run the operational side and other organs and glands to participate in the processing.

This knock-on effect can then create general symptoms, such as fatigue, in addition to localized ones such as bloating, bowel irregularities and abdominal pain. Unfortunately, all this negativity is likely to encourage the sufferer to comfort eating and reduce their activity, adding to the initial problem – and so it goes on. Often the benefit people experience as a result of giving up or cutting down on certain foods is due not only to giving their digestive system a chance to clear itself out, but because they introduce food sources that contain nutrients they had been missing out on.

How Tough Is Your Gut?

When we eat we are allowing external substances to pass into the internal world of the body – after all the body must have essential resources in the form of nutrients to keep it functioning. However, this invariably means ingesting potentially dangerous or damaging elements that come as part and parcel of the food source or attached to it, for instance in the form of bacteria. The gut is therefore heavily guarded by the immune system and protected by a strong cellular wall. The gut wall needs to be very strong to prevent harmful elements passing through but it also needs to be porous so that essential nutrients can filter into the system. In theory, in order for nutrients to pass through the gut wall, food must be broken up into minute particles. A healthy digestive system does this by subjecting it to powerful stomach acids and bacteria, and mechanically churning it and breaking it down as it moves through the system.

If the permeability of the gut wall is as it should be, then only small particles can pass through and the immune system will be ready and waiting on the other side of the wall just in case anything harmful does pass through. To stop the immune response reacting to nutrients as they pass through, and to stop it from reacting to every little tiny thing that sneaks into the body, the body has devised a system of recognition. The immune system is set up to react to alien elements over a certain size. This allows the small particles of nutrients to pass harmlessly into the body but enables the immune system to respond to the presence of larger molecules such as bacteria, a virus or unprocessed waste. This recognition process means that small particles of essential nutrients can pass into the body without creating an immune reaction, whereas larger harmful particles cannot and if they do, they become accountable to the immune system. This is a very efficient and logical process – so why do so many people have trouble with their digestive systems?

Excessive or prolonged stress, coupled with unhealthy lifestyle practices and poor diet, have the same effect on the digestive system as anywhere else in the body. The digestive system is powered by muscular action so wasting and fatigue will slow the system down and reduce its effectiveness. The digestive system is controlled by the brain and any instructions it sends out will also become slow, and possibly inaccurate, leading to dysfunctional processing. The digestive system is also a cellular structure and hence it suffers from the damaging effects of oxidation and toxins. Unfortunately, as cells weaken and energy and nutritional supplies drop, mistakes occur and a backlog of jobs builds up. As a result, a gulf emerges between the amount of work required to rectify the growing problems and continue effective functioning, and the amount of resources and ability available to do the job.

Starving The System

Already, a simple lack of power has resulted in the digestive system becoming dysfunctional. In a healthy system, any food ingested will be completely processed so that every available beneficial nutrient is obtained from it and utilized in the body. An unhealthy system will have less capacity to process foods effectively and so less nutritional value will be obtained from them. Not only does this mean that the body will receive less of the essential nutrients it so desperately needs but it will also generate more waste in the gut, slowing the system down even more and decreasing energy levels still further. This makes you more inclined to reach for a stimulant, such as alcohol or caffeine, to boost energy levels but unfortunately this adds to the waste, toxin and chemical build-up in the system, draining it yet again. An increase in toxins and stimulants also means an increase in acid levels. This not only causes people to suck away on antacid tablets, but can encourage or increase the symptoms of a whole range of conditions such as cystitis and arthritis.

Bacteria also thrive in an acid environment, piling more work onto your immune system. The gut contains numerous bacteria – many of these aid digestion and absorption, while others are a by product of food. In a healthy gut, bacteria is controlled at a safe level, while allowing it to get on with the job of keeping the digestive tract healthy. However, a combination of high acids, low energy, poor processing and high levels of sugar and yeast-based foods in the diet causes bacteria to multiply excessively in the gut thus producing abdominal bloating, pain and yeast-based infections such as thrush. These harmful bacteria can also damage the walls of the gut and this, combined with the weakening effects of oxidation and toxins, can produce a condition known as leaky gut.

Food Intolerance

Leaky gut occurs when the permeability of the gut wall has increased to an unhealthy level. This can happen as a result of injury or illness but more commonly it is caused by a slow process of digestive decline. A highly permeable gut wall allows harmful substances such as acid and bacteria to pass into the rest of the body. The gut is designed to tolerate these things but other systems are not and hence this can lead to health problems, pain and fatigue.

A leaky gut will also allow ineffectively processed food particles to pass through the gut wall. This generates two main problems. First, because these large particles are unprocessed, they are unusable and simply become a bit of waste that has provided no nutritional benefit. Secondly, because they are large, they are likely to trigger off an immune reaction. This reaction is then memorized by the immune system, which categorizes the food as a harmful substance. Your body has now developed an intolerance to that particular food because if you eat it again, your immune response will remember that it is harmful and react accordingly.

A food intolerance is therefore an inappropriate immune reaction to a food source, the usual cause of which is ineffectively processed food passing through the gut wall. Your immune system reacts to this unprocessed food by generating an inflammatory response, creating swelling and pain. Unlike an allergy, where reactions occur as soon as you come into contact with the food, symptoms of an intolerance could take hours or even days to occur as the food has to pass through the digestive system first. Some foods take up to five days to process and this makes it very difficult to identify the offending food – or to even consider food as the problem. Another difficulty with detection stems from the fact that the foods that are creating the problem are often those you enjoy or eat the most. If you eat a lot of the same foods, this increases the chance of a reaction to them. However, your immune system, as well as your taste buds, can encourage you to eat more of these foods. This occurs because when the immune response is triggered it also sets off the stress response to help the body solve the problem. When the stress response is activated, you will get an adrenaline rush that instigates anti-inflammatory and pain-killing forces, followed by a few pleasure stimuli – just as you would with any other stress response. This is known as masking and even though this feel-good factor is short-lived and the long-term negative symptoms soon kick in, it is still enough to give you a small window of relief. This then encourages you to continue eating it, which, of course, results in chronic problems such as fatigue, bloating, weight gain, IBS, inflammation and pain, because your system is never free of the offending food.

Tackling a food intolerance can dramatically improve your health but you need to look at the complete picture if you want to maintain that health, recover from your intolerance and avoid further intolerant reactions. It is very tricky to identify which food is at the root of any intolerance – especially with so many poor methods of testing available – so to get the best results you need to look at your whole diet and lifestyle. There is no point following an elimination diet in the hope it will solve your fatigue problems for example, if you are still eating three bars of chocolate, drinking ten cups of coffee and smoking 20 cigarettes a day. You need to tackle all the elements that are adversely affecting your health. An excessive intake of sugar, for example, can create a tremendous amount of strain on your body – despite the fact that it is the only food you cannot be biologically intolerant to. This is because it does not contain a protein and it is the proteins in food that trigger an immune response. Sugar may not contain protein, so technically you cannot be intolerant to it, but it can still have a more detrimental effect on health than an intolerance.

What's Your Poison?

Diets that contain an excessive amount of particular types of food can give your digestive system problems so examine your diet and see what you OD on.

- Foods that bacteria thrive off:
  Sugar – found, for instance, in cakes, chocolate, biscuits, honey, fruit, fizzy drinks and puddings.
  Yeast – found in many foods, including bread, buns, cheese, alcohol and mushrooms.
  The symptoms of a bacterial imbalance include thrush, cystitis, IBS, abdominal bloating, fungal infections, fatigue, poor concentration and brain 'fogginess'.
- Foods that are acidic:
  Fruit, yeast, sugar, cheese, coffee, fizzy drinks and alcohol.
  The symptoms of an acid imbalance include stomach ulcers, burning stomach pains, acid flow back, painful joints and muscles, lower back pains, burning sensations in the bladder, headaches and, of course, fatigue.
- Foods that are most likely to generate sensitivity:
  Wheat, dairy produce, citrus fruit, tomatoes, seafood, sugar and processed foods.
  Symptoms of a food sensitivity include migraines or sudden headaches, fatigue after eating, bloating, abdominal pains and skin rashes.
- Foods most likely to generate an intolerance:
  Wheat, dairy produce and yeast-based foods.
  The symptoms of a food intolerance can appear as chronic conditions such as IBS, ME, eczema, dermatitis, dry or flaky skin, migraines or persistent headaches, and chronic fatigue.
- Foods you are most likely to crave:
  Yeast-based foods and sugary, salty, high-calorie, processed and fatty foods.

The symptoms of an excess intake of such foods include sudden drops and fluctuations in energy, weak muscles, joint stiffness, poor skin quality and appearance, bladder or abdominal discomfort, PMT, thrush, gynaecological pains, loss in concentration and nerve sensitivity.

- Substances that stimulate:
  Nicotine, alcohol, anything containing caffeine (tea, coffee, fizzy drinks etc.), sugar and salt.
  The symptoms of an excessive stimulant intake include palpitations, chest pains, inflamed skin, sore muscles and joints, bladder and digestive irregularities, emotional and hormonal imbalances and insomnia.

Look For The Signs

Negative responses to food are there to tell you that something does not suit you. One of the greatest things about finally getting to grips with my diet was losing all those emotional hang-ups that we often associate with eating. Now my body is in balance, I look forward to eating but have lost my constant craving and compulsion for food. I have lost my addiction to certain foods, thrown out my scales, balanced my weight and developed a rational attitude to my body image. Once I had addressed the physical imbalances, I didn't need to address the psychological issues because they had disappeared naturally. My body had no reason to cause me any more hang-ups because I was feeding it with what it wanted. You may not believe me but I went from confirmed chocoholic to a complete disinterest in it – it is not a chore for me to not eat it, I simply don't want to. If I get run down, overdo things or just feel hungry, the foods I now crave are things like broccoli and parsnips! I love to eat healthy foods because they make me feel and look good and I love the taste. If a food makes you feel healthy and you enjoy the taste this is the most obvious sign that it is doing your body good. In contrast, if you suffer from a chronic condition, fatigue or have an emotional conflict with food then your diet is not working well for you.

Long-Term Relief

When you are assessing your symptoms, you need to look at the consistency of your health and be wary of things that give you short-term relief, as these may well be causing your problems or adding to them. Unfortunately, our lifestyles today tend to encourage us to take the quick-fix option rather than considering our overall long-term health and well-being. Highly stimulating foods such as sugar and chemical stimulants such as caffeine can become compulsive because of their ability to initiate stimulation. We have already looked at how your body can become dependent on foods that give an instant energy boost but the problem is compounded by the fact that the more your body becomes dependent on immediate energy sources or stimulants, the more it will demand them. This can lead to energy problems, constant hunger, cravings and weight issues.

It's easy to see why some foods generate stimulation – they are high in glucose or fat, making it easier for your body to provide a quick release of energy. The foods you are most likely to crave are foods that are capable of producing higher amounts of immediate energy – the higher the calorie content, the bigger the energy rush and the faster the satisfaction. This is why we love foods that are high in sugar and fat, like chocolate, cheese and deep-fried meals. For the body, they are some of the purest forms of energy supplies so processing is quick. This means that when they are eaten, they flood the body with a rush of new energy that the body finds very satisfying. They also trigger off the stress response, giving the body a sudden rush of adrenaline. This is why we like them so much more than lettuce and why we miss them so much if we try to deprive ourselves of them without addressing the reason why we have become dependent on them.

However, it is wrong to label foods such as chocolate and chips as 'bad' items that need be permanently excluded from the diet if they cause you no adverse effects and you follow the golden rule of not overdosing on them. If you think back to how the body likes to be run, you will remember it needs to experience positive stimulation on a daily basis. Well, food is part of that pleasure. For example, apparently chocolate releases the same pleasure stimuli as those released during sex (although you could say that chocolate is a lot more reliable and easier to get your hands on!). A healthy, balanced body likes to experience stimulation from a whole array of different things and it treats the satisfaction it gets from food as a part of that because it is an essential requirement. Enjoying your food is a healthy response but craving and over-eating things that ultimately damage your health is not. If you have a balanced body and you experience satisfaction and pleasure from living, you will enjoy the odd bowl of chips, piece of chocolate or glass of wine and be satisfied with it. When people are not satisfied by the occasional indulgence, it is often a reflection of a general dissatisfaction they feel with their lives. In such cases, food can offer a readily available source of satisfaction – and distraction. Okay so chocolate may well make a good substitute for a decent relationship for a while but there's a price – you'll need to eat a hell of a lot of it, which of course will probably just make you fat and generate a whole new set of problems. To overcome food cravings and the need for quick fixes you need to find out what drives you to depend on highly stimulating foods.

Don't forget we are looking at a symptom of an imbalance. Highly stimulating foods become a prop if you use them to try and boost flagging energy levels caused by over-stimulation, or as a means of experiencing pleasure and satisfaction because your life is lacking in positive stimulation. If your body is continuously undernourished and over-stressed it will crave these foods sources in a desperate attempt to boost energy levels. Similarly, if you have ongoing emotional anxieties and very little satisfaction in your life, these foods can become your main source of comfort and satisfaction. The addictive element derives from the fact that these foods are converted very quickly into energy – but this immediate boost will be short-lived and will, in a very short space of time, leave you tired and miserable again. The rapid return of negative symptoms, combined with the additional strain of dealing with the aftermath of sudden stimulation, sends signals out to the brain that your body does not want to feel like this, it would like to feel like it did half an hour ago when it was stimulated. This instigates a craving for more of the stimulant – be it chocolate or cheese – and this constant craving can lead to addiction.

In a healthy body, stimulants such as chocolate can be easily dealt with, allowing you to experience the pleasure without the strain. However, most people who crave stimulating substances feel the need for them because they are unhappy or tired. If your body is already run down and operating ineffectively then constant exposure to anything over-stimulating and lacking in nourishment will put a further strain on energy supplies and resources. It requires a great deal of effort for a weakened system to deal with sudden stimulation.

The Effect Of Stimulants

It is not just high-glucose and high-fat foods that can stimulate. Foods high in acid, salt and yeast can, in excess, over-stimulate the body and generate cravings. Alcohol, caffeine, nicotine and other natural and chemical stimulants have all been turned into user-friendly concoctions that extract the maximum buzz out of them. Alcohol, caffeine and nicotine are in fact relaxants but they stimulate the body by triggering the stress response. They do this by rapidly upsetting the natural balance of the body – they produce a very immediate and deep relaxation that panics the body into producing an immediate rush of stimulation to counter-balance the effects of the relaxation. The body feels that if this very deep and immediate relaxation is not rectified then it could 'shut down', so it acts by instigating a stress response that floods the body with adrenaline to get it moving again. This is why you may have a glass of wine, cigarette or cup of tea as a means to relax after a busy day or after a traumatic event but you also use them as a stimulant to 'get the party going' or to make you feel more alert.

The problem with the body instigating emergency action is that it tends to overcompensate in an attempt to put things right. If you kick a bucket of water, the water has to slosh about before it can settle again. The harder the kick, the longer it takes to settle. This is similar to how your body deals with imbalances. The bigger and more urgent the imbalance, the greater the action of the body, which swings from one extreme to another before settling. Extreme or continual use of these stimulants will throw your system into one imbalance after another, putting a further strain on your energy, resources and cellular structure.

Nicotine, caffeine and other chemically produced substances are often referred to as toxic because they create additional toxicity in the body. As we have seen, the manufacture of energy also produces toxins, so the body already has the capacity to remove toxins. This is why a healthy system can cope with exposure to the odd toxin but cannot cope with constant exposure – for a dysfunctional system this sort of exposure is particularly harmful.

One of the ways that toxins such as nicotine and caffeine stimulate the body is by scaring it into action. Remember, there is a set procedure to the stress response that starts with an adrenaline rush, whether the prompt is pleasurable or life-threatening. The body holds a supply of energy for times of emergency. This is why we can go to bed absolutely exhausted but be wide awake and running away from danger at the merest sound of something sinister.

Addiction Chart

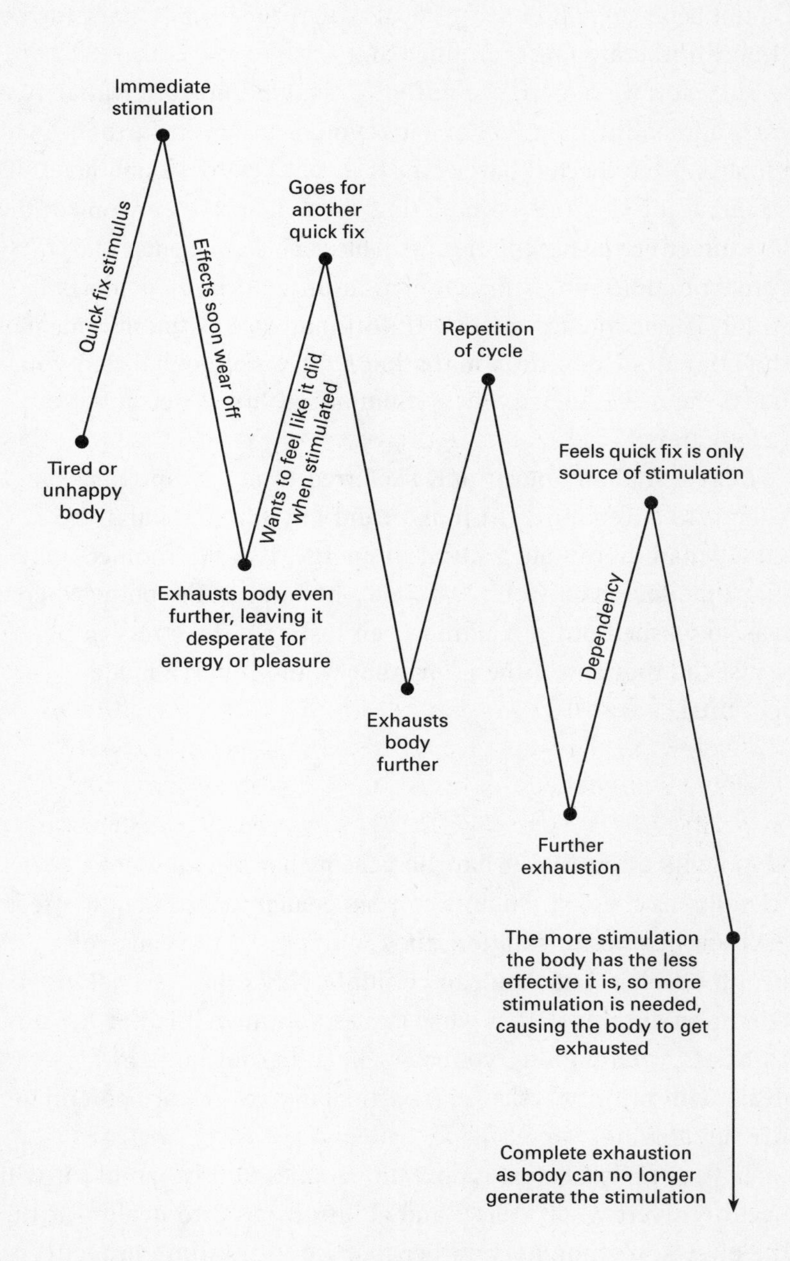

The same thing happens in the body when you take in toxic substances. As soon as the substance enters your system, your body has to activate itself to deal with a potentially harmful, even life-threatening substance and this generates the stimulation we experience during consumption. Unfortunately, each adrenaline rush will exhaust your body even further, making it harder and harder for it to produce the same level of stimulation. The more stimulating substances are consumed, the less effective the stimulation becomes. This is because the constant additional stress and strain on your body depletes its supply of emergency energy. Unfortunately, low energy makes the body desperate for stimulation so the more exhausted your body, the more addictive the stimulant – thus it becomes your energy 'prop'.

When my body burnt out, I referred to my symptoms as an allergy to adrenaline. If I took or did anything stimulating, rather than giving me a boost of energy, it would immediately make me feel even worse. My body had got to the point where it was so washed out it couldn't even instigate the stress response – just the thought of the effort that would involve made it feel tired.

Chronic Conditions

My clients often find it hard to accept that something as 'society friendly' as these stimulants can have such a detrimental effect on their health. In isolation, they may not be the cause of a health problem but they can certainly play a part in making a condition chronic. Often what makes you unwell is not the same as what is maintaining your poor health. Your body always deals with priority tasks first, particularly if they are potentially life threatening.

If your body is already low on supplies and capability it will need to divert what energy and ability it has into dealing with the effects of stimulants, rather than concentrating on recovery and renewal. If you cause unnecessary and additional strain on your body by putting in things that create more work for it, it will need to use what little reserves it has to deal with these additional problems, rather than using them to improve your health and energy levels. The weaker your system the less it will be able to tolerate anything that causes additional strain. I can't begin to think how many times I have heard people say, 'Well it can't be that because I have been doing it for years and never had a problem with it before.'

It can be hard to comprehend that something you have done for years could be a component in your current health problems but you must never assume that what you did to your body when you were healthy and happy will be okay to do when you are unhealthy or unhappy. You can get away with a lot when you have a healthy, happy body – when you don't, you need to give it additional care and consideration.

Wonderful Water

In addition to essential nutrients, you need to put fluid into your system and the only fluid your body really needs is water. Okay so it may be dull compared to a pina colada or triple espresso but you cannot survive without it. Countless people are suffering from fatigue and health problems simply because they do not drink enough, or even any, pure water. Seventy per cent of your body is made up of water – not cola, coffee or gin and tonic – and it needs to be constantly replaced as it is used up or becomes polluted. Water is an essential multi-tasker. Amongst other things it transports nutrients and energy supplies, flushes out waste and toxins, acts as a suspending agent to allow bodily processes to occur, provides form and structure and helps control blood pressure.

To get the most benefit from water it needs to be in its pure form. If you add things they can change its properties, making it harder to utilize or completely useless. For example, caffeine or alcohol act as a diuretic, which means that they flush fluid out of the body, leading to dehydration and toxicity. Your body contains miles of pipe work to enable it to transport resources and energy to every extremity and to remove potentially damaging substances and toxins from the system. Water in the body works like water in a hosepipe. A strong, steady flow of water will provide enough force to get the water right to the end of the pipe and keep the pipe clear of debris. If there is only a trickle of water in the pipe, then distribution slows down and residue will collect along the length of the pipe.

Fluid Retention

Pressure of fluid also dictates your blood pressure. If your blood pressure is too low you become lethargic; too much pressure and your energy may well be high initially but everything will soon begin to get worn out. When your body is stimulated, adrenaline forces your blood pressure up and one of the ways it does this is by retaining more fluid. Sodium plays a vital role in this process as it controls the retention of fluid in the body. When you are stimulated, your body retains and utilizes sodium to force the pressure of fluid up. Foods high in salt have the same effect because they stimulate the body by increasing your saline levels thereby pushing up internal fluid pressure. If you have had a prolonged period of stress or anxiety then fluid can build up, resulting in problems such as bloating, inflammation, weight gain and fatigue. When you then relax, you may find that you need to pee more because the body wants to relieve itself of additional fluid and the toxins it contains.

This example demonstrates why it is so important to take an integrated approach if you want to improve your health and well-being. You do need to put the right things in but you also need to make sure you are creating the right environment to enable your body to utilize all those nutrients effectively. An imbalance in your lifestyle can lead to a poor supply of essential supplies, no matter how healthy your diet appears to be. A healthy diet is no good in isolation; it will help but your best results will come from combining it with a healthy approach to living.

Good Nutrition, Good News

The good news is that you can reverse the process of poor health through poor nutrition. The first step is to find out which foods suit you. Symptoms such as fatigue, dramatic daily slumps in energy, weight problems, bloating, fluid retention, digestive disorders and chronic conditions can all be related back to what you do and don't put into your body. We have looked at a whole combination of reasons why what you put into your body can affect the health of it, but how do you start to discover which foods are best for *you*?

I encourage my clients to start off with a basic diet containing the foods most likely to provide good nutrition and least likely to cause a negative response. Even so, this is not guaranteed and the safest and most effective way of discovering your own perfect diet is to continually assess your progress. I like to start my clients off with a simple 14-day diet and then continuously assess and review so that they can decide what to incorporate over the next 14-day stage and so on. This means that they can start to reintroduce foods or address negative responses at various stages throughout the process. Cutting out a food for a short period of time has very few disadvantages but could still give you time to detect if there is any improvement in health or a negative reaction. I don't like to count calories or get too bogged down with quantities because we often don't realize how much we should and can eat of the right foods. There is a misconception that because we need to limit our intake of so-called 'bad' foods, we need to limit our intake of all types of foods.

The foods I include in the first stage of the 14-day diet are what I call basic food sources. This means meat, fish and vegetables, for instance, rather than a whole plethora of ingredients that have been lumped together with additives and chemicals to form a ready-meal. Many of the foods included are simple foods that cause least strain on the body – foods that are easy for the body to process so that you can reduce the amount of stress on your digestive system. These foods are also the least likely to generate an intolerant reaction, sensitivity, excessive stimulation or bloating and are as near as possible to the foods the body was designed to eat when it was put together all those millions of years ago.

This diet works particularly well for those suffering from stress-related conditions like fatigue and weight problems, as it is designed to increase energy levels. I always like to initially concentrate on improving energy because once levels start to rise, the body can then deal more effectively with other emotional and physical symptoms. If I was seeing someone individually, I would consider if this advice was relevant to them but, from a general perspective, it has proven to be very effective – and I say that from personal, as well as professional, experience. It is the diet that I put together; the one that kick-started my route to recovery. Of course everyone is different, which is why I only like people to try it for a short period and continually update and assess the results. The result you get, whether negative or positive, will dictate the direction you take so see this as the starting point to uncovering your own personal route to recovery.

Assess Your Results

Before we move on to the actual content of the diet it would help to explain a little bit about the possible outcome. The results of the diet will dictate your next step so you need to constantly assess and reassess because only through this process of change will you determine what does and does not work for you as an individual.

There are three potential results:

1. Good – this means any change that can be seen as an improvement.
2. No change – there are no effects whatsoever.
3. Not good – anything that gives overall negative results.

If Your Results Are Good

If you are feeling better, livelier, slimmer or fitter for example, even if only slightly, then the diet is obviously working. This is great but you need to decide on your next step so that you can sustain the positive result and even improve on it.

Things to consider

- Do you want to start reintroducing foods?
  You may want to carry on with the diet as it is until you have reached your health goal before thinking about expanding your diet to form an eating plan that suits your life. Alternatively, you may find that you are struggling with the restrictions and need to reintroduce some items to make it easier to continue. If reintroducing items results in a decline in health then at least you will be aware that what you have reintroduced is generating negative responses. However, to be able to isolate the cause of the problem, you will need to reintroduce foods gradually. This allows you to assess how they are affecting you and exactly what is causing the negative symptoms.
- Can you do anything else to increase your success?
  Combining your new diet plan with changes in lifestyle will give you the greatest chance of success in the fastest possible time. If you want to speed up your progress, check if you are still doing anything that could still be putting a strain on

your body, and also if there is anything beneficial that you could now introduce into your plan. You also need to be aware of any new negative responses, no matter how small, or any change in the intensity of existing problems. When you make positive changes, there could still be some negative effects, for example you may suffer from feelings of deprivation because something pleasurable has been removed from your life or you may find the reaction of other people is not as supportive as you would have liked. It is important that you are aware that these negative elements could occur. You can then limit their effect on your progress by focusing on your overall success and not any minor irritations that crop up along the way.

If You Experience No Change

Remember, it has probably taken a long time to become as tired, unhappy or run down as you may be feeling now so it could take time to see any progress.

Things to consider

- You may not have been doing the diet for long enough. It can take up to six months for some people to see real progress, which is why you need to assess and review continuously.
- Are you being strict enough? We all know that it is very easy to give in to our cravings, particularly at the beginning of a diet when the body is adjusting to a new way of eating. You need to ensure you are really sticking to the eating plan because, at this early stage, just one indulgence could make a difference if your system is very sensitive. You are the one that will benefit from the change so make sure you are really giving your body the opportunity to experience that benefit.
- Something you are still eating may be causing an adverse effect. If you have been strictly adhering to the diet and you are not getting any positive results then one of the foods on the diet could be affecting you. Having pared your diet down

to basic food items, it will be easier for you now to locate what the culprit is. This means that you need to concentrate your detective powers on what you are still eating as one of those items could be irritating your system.

- You have not introduced your new diet plan in conjunction with healthy changes to your lifestyle. If your body is still under constant stress it will find it hard to take advantage of the improved nutritional supply.
- Your body does not like the way you are serving your food. For example, some people have problems eating raw food but have no problems eating the same food if it is cooked; others find that food cooked in fat upsets their system. Try changing the way you prepare your food – it might just make a difference.

If You Are Having Bad Results

Firstly, do bear in mind that for the first few days you may experience minor negative reactions as your body starts to detox and adjust. You may well feel more tired, get a headache or experience minor skin reactions. However, this is to be expected and should pass in a few days.

If your symptoms are serious or they persist, you should stop immediately and go back to your normal diet – I also recommend you see your doctor. I have to stress that this sort of reaction happens very, very rarely but it does happen so you need to be aware of it. You may simply have an illness or virus whose appearance at this particular time is coincidental, or it may be that something in the diet is seriously irritating your body. The diet contains foods that the average body favours, therefore if you are experiencing an adverse reaction you do not have an average body. This could happen if you changed your diet in any way, not just as a result of this diet. An adverse reaction may not be the result you were hoping for but it is still a result. You can learn from negative reactions, just as you can learn from positive ones.

If you get an adverse reaction from eating what should be perfectly harmless foods then you have, and probably always have had, a serious sensitivity to one of those foods. Things like this often only come to light because a change in diet has meant you are eating more of this food. For example, you may be intolerant to eggs but because you have only eaten them as an ingredient, the level of consumption has been so low as to cause only a minor reaction like a headache or drop in energy – the sort of reaction that you could put down to anything. This is what I mean by positive results – even if the initial effects are not necessarily good you are still taking a step toward discovering the cause of your ill health. If you have an intolerance to a certain food and changing to a healthier diet increases your reaction to that intolerance then the stronger adverse reaction and limited food range should make it easier to pinpoint the cause of the problem – and an intolerance test or following a process of elimination could soon clarify your suspicions.

That initial unpleasant reaction could be the catalyst for a dramatic improvement in your overall health because it enabled you to isolate the cause and deal with it once and for all. Success comes from knowing what steps to take with every assessment you make along the way. Theoretically, no one should experience problems as a result of eating healthy food but in reality a small percentage will. If you are aware of that possibility and know how to act then the overall result for you in the long run could be very positive. Certainly, anyone reacting badly to healthy food should seriously consider having a food intolerance test. This is why I strongly suggest you get the support of health professionals, particularly your doctor, to provide reassurance throughout your journey to recovery. The information I give you here is only a guide to what *could* work, as is the information given by any other health professional. It may seem that there are endless and conflicting views available but this also means you have a wide range of options to choose from. The final choice and responsibility lies with you and this is why it is so important to understand your body. The more you know about how it likes to be run and the sort of resources it requires, the easier it will be for you to make your own educated choices about health. Rather than seeing the vast range of health advice as bewildering, you will be able to select what you know will have a good chance of success and disregard the less credible options.

Starting Point Programme

This basic diet will help restore energy and health.

This is your permitted list of foods for the first 14 days:
Meat – any meat, for instance beef, lamb, pork, ham, bacon, chicken, turkey, game, duck and goose.
Fish and seafood – all fish and seafood, for instance white fish, tuna, mackerel, sardines, salmon, swordfish, prawns, mussels and squid.
Vegetables – all vegetables except onions, mushrooms and tomatoes, which are technically a fruit but some people class them as a vegetable. Permitted vegetables include potatoes, parsnips, carrots, green vegetables, beans and peppers.
Eggs
Rice
Nuts – all nuts, for instance hazelnuts, almonds, peanuts and pecans
Seeds – all seeds, for instance sunflower and pumpkin
Pulses – lentils and all the beans such as kidney and black eye
Drink – water only

DON'T EAT ANYTHING THAT YOU KNOW YOU ALREADY REACT TO, DON'T LIKE EATING OR DON'T EAT FOR MORAL OR RELIGIOUS REASONS.

You can eat anything that is on this list; if it is not on the list, don't eat it. On first glance the diet may seem limiting but in fact these basic food sources create the bulk of most meals, just without the trimmings of added chemicals, high stimulants and the complex processing of ready meals and snack foods.

There are no real quantity restrictions – but remember the golden rule that excessive amounts of anything can be detrimental. There is also no need to avoid fat, as long as it is part and parcel of something on the list. You can have oil, for instance, provided it is derived from sunflower seeds, peanuts etc. You can still have something you may well have always liked, like a good old roast dinner for instance, because you can have roast beef, potatoes and vegetables. I hate all those diets that involve eating plans where you have to measure quantities out or make specific meals on specific days. If you have a list of ingredient, then you can create the food you like to eat and eat it when you want to eat it.

Obviously you will need to use the list to suit your demands – for instance, if you are a vegetarian, meat is out but it is important that you have plenty of protein in non-animal forms such as nuts.

MAKE SURE YOU KEEP IT AS VARIED AND BALANCED AS POSSIBLE.

Don't get bogged down with eating the same foods at the same time every day. Make sure you vary what you have for breakfast, lunch and dinner.

Follow the diet for 14 days – provided you do not get any adverse effects – and try to stick to three good meals a day.

Preparation

Before you even attempt to begin changing your diet, you first need to check with a health professional that you are in a fit state to start your new diet and that nothing it contains could aggravate any existing health conditions.

You then need to work out how you are going to succeed by addressing where you could fail. Planning a week or so ahead before you start can increase your chances of success dramatically. Think about the foods that are available and what you want to make. You may also want to clear out your existing food stock before you feel ready to start.

Make sure you do not begin the diet until you feel confident that you know what you are doing. Start it when the time is right for you, rather than throwing yourself at the earliest possible moment. Remember that you might feel a bit groggy initially so it could help to keep a few days free at the beginning to make this period easy to cope with.

Points You Need To Consider

- Do you view this diet as restrictive?
  If so, take a trip to your local supermarket and health food shop and look at the vast array of foods you can eat. Start reading ingredients labels. A golden rule is if there are more than three ingredients on a food label, don't buy it. In fact the best foods are the ones that are so pure they don't need an ingredients label.
- Do you think that you will feel deprived?
  Look at what you can eat on the list rather than what you cannot. There are some pleasure fixes in there: for example, technically you can eat chips, as long as they are just oil and potato, simply remember the golden rule that excessive or constant intake causes harm. Also, there are lots of natural versions available of well-known processed foods. Take peanut butter as an example: mass-produced peanut butter can have lots of sugar and additives in it, whereas organic peanut butter just contains peanuts and oil and is a great source of nutrients.

- Do you think you will be tempted to stray from the diet?
Of course you will, so address temptation now to avoid failure. Ensure your house is stocked up with the right food and plan some ideas for meals. Again, look at what you can eat, rather than what you cannot. For example, for breakfast you could have bacon and eggs or rice cakes with peanut butter and for lunch you could have a baked potato with salad and prawns. Get plenty of menus sorted beforehand.
It's better if you can stick to regular meal times but if you need a snack then have some healthy nibbles around for the times when you are most likely to indulge. Take bags of nuts, seeds or raw vegetable sticks with you in the car or to work and always make sure you have plenty of water available. If you get peckish have a drink and a rest first because often your body confuses a need for water and rest with hunger.
- Do you think the diet will involve more time in food preparation and cooking?
This isn't necessarily the case – how much effort does it take to put a piece of salmon under the grill and some ready-prepared vegetables on to cook? There are many quick and easy ways of preparing simple food, and things like frozen and canned produce and slow cookers make it even easier. It is also a diet that the whole family can get involved with, so there should be no need to prepare one meal for yourself and another for everyone else. If you can get the family to eat more pure foods, rather than a diet of processed and unhealthy food, you can all become healthier together.

You have probably been eating a limited diet for a long time and have got into the habit of buying and eating the same things over the years, but if you open your eyes and start experimenting with things you don't normally eat you will discover a whole range of delicious, interesting foods that will help you on the road to a healthier body.

The Next Stage

This is where you begin your own personal process of discovery. I can start you off with a basic diet but after 14 days you need to make an assessment of how well it is working for you so that you can set yourself a diet plan for the next 14 days and so on. If the diet is going well you may consider continuing as you are or think about reintroducing other nutritious foods like fruit, milk and basic cereals over time so that you can build yourself a healthy eating plan for life.

The foods you need to consider reintroducing first are skimmed milk, fruit and cereals. When you are ready to start reintroducing foods, then add one of these food types, one at a time over a four-day period. If there are no ill effects after a week, then try reintroducing another. If any adverse effects do arise, you could have located an offending food. Leave it out of your diet for now and try reintroducing it at a later date as your body may well just be still too weak to tolerate it.

Once you have reintroduced all the foods you want to and you are feeling happier and healthier, the diet you have devised will become the basis of your maintenance eating plan. You can then consider if you want to have the odd indulgence, such as chocolate or alcohol, but you will probably find that you do not enjoy them as much as you used to and will be less inclined to overdo it. If you do indulge and experience some adverse effects as a result, you need to return to your maintenance plan.

If you are restored to near full health you can enjoy a wider diet but you may like to use your recovery diet to detox every one or two days a week. It is also helpful to return to it when you feel unwell or have health problems – at these times it will allow the body to channel more resources towards getting better. You will find out what suits your health and happiness over time, as your confidence in running your own body grows.

Eliminating The Suspects

If, as happens on rare occasions, the results are not so favourable, this is an indication that one of the foods you are still eating could be a source of irritation to you. Your next step will be to detect which food it is. Elimination diets take time so you may consider starting with an intolerance test. It is tricky to get a reliable intolerance test done, so it is best to contact a professional body like the British Allergy Foundation or see the resources page at the back of the book.

If you want to try an elimination diet, and you have already established that one of the foods you are reacting to is most likely to be from the Starting Point diet, then start by reintroducing dairy, cereals and fruit. You need to do this because if you remove food sources (i.e. the suspect foods) out of an already-restricted diet you will end up with nothing to eat. If this reintroduction does not cause any adverse effects, concentrate on those food items in the starting point diet. Take each food or food group, such as eggs or seafood, out of your diet one at a time for a maximum of 14 days. It will be pretty evident early on if your adverse reactions are still there, which will indicate that you are still eating the offending food. In this case, reintroduce the food you have eliminated and take out another. It may be the case that more than one food is responsible for your symptoms. Eventually you should see some progress. It may take time but you have probably had this problem for years, if not most of your life, and this initial effort could give you good health for the rest of it.

A Balanced Diet

The Starting Point Programme should give you a balanced diet and has the ability to give you all the nutrients your body needs

– but only if you eat a wide variety of the foods listed. For example, you need to eat plenty of vegetables to get loads of beneficial vitamins and minerals, therefore you can't just eat potatoes for two weeks. I am always reluctant to exclude dairy produce, cereals and fruit because they are extremely nutritious but in a run-down system they are also the most likely irritants. I like to keep diet restrictions to a short time-frame of 14-day periods so that as soon as your health returns you can move on to a balanced maintenance diet. During those initial recovery periods you need to look at other less traditional ways of getting the nutrients these excluded food items supply. For example, there are lots of other sources of calcium in the diet apart from dairy produce – for instance, almonds, fish, leafy green vegetables and broccoli. And if you discover that you feel better avoiding dairy produce, consider reducing your intake, have days off eating it or try finding out if it is one type of food in the group – like cheese for example – rather than excluding all dairy produce. Alternatively, permanently substitute with alternative sources of calcium already mentioned (they're wonderfully healthy anyway).

Supplements

I know there is a lot of conflicting advice about supplements and it is true that if you have a balanced diet you really should not need them. However, even if you have a healthy diet, on a daily basis can you guarantee that it is always balanced? I recommend taking supplements – as long as they are not full of all the things you are trying to avoid, like sugar and additives. There are so many types and mixes available but all I feel you need is one complete mineral and vitamin combination tablet a day and an additional calcium supplement, particularly in the initial starting point stage of your plan, just to be sure your intake is maintained. Even the most health-aware person has imbalances in their diet from day to day and if you can take something to ensure that you are getting all the nutrients you need, then why not?

Do remember, though, that just because something is healthy it doesn't mean the more you have the better – an excess of some vitamins and minerals can be harmful. However, one multivitamin tablet a day is very, very unlikely to overdose your body as the amounts needed to achieve overload are much higher than the recommended daily allowances set by a dietary committee.

It's Up To You

At the end of the day it is all down to choice, your own personal choice. You can be as strict or as lax as you wish but, if you want results in the fastest possible time, it pays to be as strict as possible initially – otherwise you will find it hard to assess the result and know in which direction to move. If you give in or give up, the only person you are giving up on is yourself. Two weeks is not a long time and it certainly doesn't mean you can never do this or never have that. What the initial diet does is give you the opportunity to take control of the health of your body rather than your health dictating a limiting life for you. Remember, you are asking the question why, when you want to say yes, your body refuses to oblige. I can give you possible reasons why and advise on how to make your body work for you but you are the only that can make it happen, the only one that can make any plan work and the only one that can experience the positive results of your efforts. If you feed your body with what it wants and what it needs, it will be happy to say yes.

Guidelines For Good Health

KEEP IT SIMPLE: Don't make life complicated for your body. It already has to deal with the toxins and damage that are a by-product of living and could do without additional irritants that sap its energy further. Basic foods are what your body was designed to run on so don't complicate your diet with foods that have little nutritional value.

VARIETY REALLY IS THE SPICE OF LIFE: Your body needs a huge array of essential nutrients, in varying quantities, and the only way that this can be achieved is through consuming a wide range of foods. Nutrients work together so there is no point overloading on one if you don't keep up supplies of any others. Don't let your diet become monotonous – keep it varied.

WATER IS LIQUID LIFE: Three quarters of the body is made up of water and you lose about 2–3 litres a day through internal pollution and dehydration so make sure you keep your system topped up and flowing.

ADDRESS YOUR CRAVINGS: Don't use stimulants as a prop because they may well become the cause of your ill health or constantly low energy levels. Not only do stimulants put excessive stress on your body, they also act as anti-nutrients, stripping your body of the essential nutrients it so desperately needs.

COMBINE YOUR EFFORTS: Changing your diet needs to be combined with a healthy approach to all aspects of your life if you want to get maximum benefits. Remember the five-point recovery plan that incorporates dealing with stress, encouraging positive stimulation and relaxation, putting the right things in and keeping harmful things out? Keep that in mind as we move on to part two.

Now that you've seen how your body likes to be run, let's see if we can sort your mind out as well.

Part Two

changing your mind

Prepare To Make A Difference

The people I help have a diverse range of problems but generally there are two key reasons why they reach the point where they feel desperate enough to seek help. The first is a lack of understanding about how they have arrived at the situation they are in and the second is lack of preparation in their attempts to resolve their problem. In order to bring about change you need to allocate time and effort to the things that will help you make that change. Unfortunately, instead of asking ourselves fundamental questions about how we intend to make this change, and getting hold of the relevant information to help us do it, we just launch in an arbitrary fashion and hope it will all work out. It's little wonder that it often doesn't.

Thorough preparation can make a huge difference to the outcome of your attempts to change and is a big factor in whether the outcome is a success or failure.

Ask yourself the following...
What do you want to do?
Why do you want to do it?
How are you going to do it?
Is it possible?
What do you expect to get out of it?
Is it worth it?

What happens if you don't do it?
If any of your answers to these questions are negative, it is not surprising that you are having difficulty solving your problem. The next few sections will help you to answer these questions in a more constructive way and by doing so you will discover what has been stopping you in the past and how you can approach your problems in future.

Satisfying Your Needs

The first thing you need to do is establish a motive for change. Why do you want to change?

This is your incentive. For most people that incentive will be the need to experience pleasure and satisfaction, which is achieved through the positive stimulation generated when you feel happy and healthy. This is your reason for living. We, as human beings, are not very good at 'must do', but we will do things willingly to get a feel-good fix. This is why all those wonderful positive stimuli and happy hormones are so important – as a reward and a motivation to continue.

In part one we looked at how important pleasure and satisfaction is, not just to your emotional well-being but also your physical health. Everything you do stems from your fundamental need to recognize the point of living. So having fun, me time, achieving and looking for personal fulfilment are not frivolous things, they are part and parcel of wanting to stay alive.

This may all seem very selfish but we are talking about pleasure *and* satisfaction. Satisfaction may not necessarily involve a pleasurable act. It could be dealing with an unpleasant situation successfully, making the most of an unpleasant environment or helping out someone in trouble. You have a better chance of experiencing satisfaction in your life if you work and get on with other people – even when they all have different goals and objectives – because we all desire love and respect from our fellow man.

If you go back to when our species was put together, in the harsh environment of primitive man, if you weren't loved or respected, chances are you would be served up for breakfast. There was no room for anything without a use or value and if you had none, then you had a big problem. So we know it is in our interests to get on, not just because it is a calculated way to get what we want but also because good relationships bring lots of positive stimuli. Traditionally, this need for social acceptance was more relevant to women because men could gain respect from a show of physical strength and it didn't necessarily matter if that made them unpopular. Without that strength, women have had to resort more to securing their position by fulfilling others desires and wishes – which makes it harder for them to consider their own. On the positive side, this means that women are better at forming friendships whereas men can often feel unloved and isolated. Recent research at the University of Michigan showed that women who regularly helped people out were, on average, 50 per cent more likely to outlive their unhelpful counterparts.

The big dilemma we have is how to fulfil our need for pleasure and satisfaction. Most of us look to what society dictates will be most likely to bring satisfaction. Traditionally this means we spend our early adult life trying to achieve, for example, a good career, a happy family and the trappings of wealth in the hope this will bring us recognition. Then we get to our mid 30s and realize that rather than bringing satisfaction, it has made us tired and depressed. As the years roll by we become more despondent until we reach our 40s or 50s and have a major mid-life crisis. In today's society some of us are bringing our mid-life crisis forward into our 30s and even our 20s because of the speed of decline in our health and well-being. The chances of successfully changing your life if you wait until you are desperate, or are forced into it due to ill health, are very low – unless you are well prepared. When you do things out of desperation it is unlikely that you can ever have any control over the results. For a lucky few it can be fantastic throwing themselves into a dramatic life change, but if you are one of the unprepared majority this only brings more anxiety and disappointment, making you even more reluctant to attempt any further change for the better.

This is where preparation is paramount. It can help you view your options and test-run a few of them without upsetting the status quo. Then you can decide which of your choices are worth persevering with. For instance, you may discover that in fact you don't need a change of career, simply some new interests and a bigger social circle. Amateur dramatics and a weekly writing circle may not initially seem very life changing but over time they could be inspiring. You will find that you are at your most successful when you do something you are passionate about. A small but inspiring change will not only give you immediate pleasure but will encourage you to search further for overall satisfaction in other areas of your life.

Question Your Incentives

You may find it hard to implement change because you have not accurately pinpointed the cause of your problem. For example, if you think your problem is constant tiredness and you ask yourself why you are always tired, your answer will probably be along the lines of too much stress, anxiety, pressure or a heavy workload. However, if I were asking you the question, I would want to know why you had too much of these things or why your body was not coping with these perfectly normal aspects of life. Is it because you have emotional insecurities, physical weaknesses, a poor diet or lack of enjoyment in life? Your fatigue is a symptom of something and you need to discover what that something is if you are to improve your energy levels.

Your incentive is to stop feeling tired, therefore you have to accept that something in your life is making you tired and this needs to be addressed if you want to feel lively again.

Let's look at other typical *symptoms* of poor health that are often classed as the *problem*: excess weight, smoking or excessive drinking. If you see these as your problem, ask yourself why you want to give them up. You will no doubt come out with all the usual answers about feeling more confident, happier, healthier and looking better, when in fact it is the lack of these elements in your life that is making you smoke, drink or over-eat. Your excess weight, or your need to smoke or drink, is due to your lack of confidence, happiness, health and good body image – so these are the problems you should be addressing.

You need to ask yourself why you have no confidence, why your health is poor, why you have such a poor body image and why you are unhappy.

You have not been able to address these things in the past because you have been unaware of your true incentive for change. Addressing symptomatic problems alone will not necessarily make you happy or resolve the issues that started you on the path to unhealthy practices. All the problems that generated these negative symptoms will still be there.

Of course successfully dealing with these things could make you more confident, happier and healthier because it has shown you that you can achieve things and take control of your situation. However, if you do not address the initial cause, you may find the changes hard to sustain. If you were happier, healthier and in control of your life then you wouldn't have these addictions and negative symptoms – they would go away of their own accord.

In my experience, once I tackled the root cause of my ill health everything began to miraculously improve. I put up with loads of horrid little health problems for years – such as poor skin, cystitis, endometriosis, chilblains, mouth-ulcers, weight gain, bloating, aches and pains, kidney problems – but to my mind my health only became a real problem when I developed ME. If you had asked me what I wanted, I would have said more energy. So why didn't I have more energy after four years of lying around doing nothing?

The reason was that I was not addressing why I had developed the health problems that had sapped my energy. Once I dealt with my inherent weakness, prolonged stress and poor diet that were at the root of my problems my health returned better than it had ever been before. Everything negative just seemed to vanish and I was left with loads of energy, great skin, balanced weight and no aches and pains. This is what I want you to achieve. Go back to the earlier questions and have a closer look at what you really want to achieve. I am sure the answer will be that you just want to be happier – and to achieve that you need to be healthier and in control of your life, rather than your life controlling you. Your motivation for change will become much greater if your incentive is to become happier or healthier, as this will open up a whole range of new approaches and options for you to try out rather than feeling stuck with one seemingly unsolvable situation.

Look Closer At Your Incentive

When was the last time you made time to enjoy life?
Why are you unhappy now?
When was the last time you felt in control of your health?
Do you understand why you are unhealthy or unhappy?
Will your intended change make you happier or healthier?
Why will it?
What has been stopping you from improving your situation?
What do you need to deal with first?

Experiencing pleasure and satisfaction is fundamental to happy and healthy living; if they are not a part of your life then it's hardly surprising you have problems. If you do not focus on these two elements as your main incentive it will be hard to have the motivation to change. Your aim, therefore, is to find ways of encouraging them back into your life.

Ditching Disappointment

We have established that no two people are the same, so finding out what satisfies us is a matter of experience. We all have to experiment and make choices about which direction to take in life. It is this process that generates so many emotional insecurities: fear of making the wrong choice, fear of failure, inability to decide, fear of the unknown and fear of making things worse all develop as you suffer setbacks and disappointments. If your life appears to be one long series of setbacks and disappointments you will find that you deliberately start to reduce your level of experimentation because you have become tired of generating more potential problems. Although this creates a safer environment for you, it also creates one with less potential to stimulate, hence feelings of resentment and a sense of under-achievement begin to surface. If you are tired of being in that rut, you need to find a way of making positive changes without incurring another blow to your self-esteem. With preparation you can create a safe environment to experiment and discover where your source of satisfaction really lies.

Good preparation will reduce the risk of disappointment or the effects of it. When people find it hard to make a change, fear of disappointment is often at the root of it. Feelings of disappointment and dissatisfaction are there for a very good reason. Again we can trace this back, quite literally, to evolution. Basically if we didn't have the ability to experience dissatisfaction we would still be living in caves, sleeping on stone beds, eating raw meat and wearing furry hot pants.

You have to experiment to make the most of your life and feelings of disappointment are there to help you decipher what will and won't work in the future, as well as giving you the motivation to improve your situation. It is thanks to humankind's dissatisfaction that we now have electric blankets and fully fitted carpets.

Looking back to the past is a great way of reminding yourself of where your successes lie or of assessing how much you have improved your situation. However, you cannot change the past, you can only learn from it. You can use past information as a way of preparing for a better future but dwelling in the past can often create insecurities and unrealistic expectations about the future. There is only one thing you can be sure of in life and that is change. If you do not make your own decisions to change in the future then change will continue to happen but without you having a hand in it. This will lead you to fear the future, as well as experiencing dissatisfaction with your current situation.

Some of my clients have life-threatening illnesses and know that there are unpleasant things to come in the future. Quite rightly they are undergoing medical treatment for their problem but they find that this reduces their sense of control, thereby increasing their anxiety over their future. However, once they understand that they do have some element of control over their life, they find it easier to come to terms with the reality of the situation. Regaining responsibility for things like their approach to their illness, attitude, lifestyle and personal health care has often lead to a dramatic improvement in overall health and well-being. Anything you do to make life easier for your body will assist it greatly in its ability to combat disease and illness and this can make a huge difference to your chances of success. It is the same with the mind. It needs to feel that you are attempting to make positive steps to improve a situation; if you don't, it will tell you by way of negative responses.

There is no doubt that disappointment and dissatisfaction are unpleasant but if they are recognized and used in a positive way they can greatly increase your chances of getting what you want. Hindsight, apparently, is a wonderful thing but the more you prepare, the greater the chance of success – and the less you will need to learn after the event.

Which Example Will You Follow?

The following example demonstrates the difference preparation can make to an outcome.

I want you to imagine two similar, equally qualified women who have been invited to attend a job interview. They both have an equal chance of getting the job, or have they?

The first one feels there is no point in putting in much preparation because she knows that, on paper, she has a good chance of success. Her attitude is very positive because she believes she is so well qualified that her risk of disappointment is low and this fills her with confidence. She has spent the night before the interview getting excited about what she will do when she gets the job and has been through a perfect scenario for the following day in her head; even working out an amusing reply in response to being offered the job on the spot.

This has left her calm and refreshed and she sleeps very well – so well, in fact, that she oversleeps, has no time to iron her shirt, then the car won't start and she arrives late. She is then asked lots of difficult questions about the job and the company that she can't answer and, by the time she leaves, she knows there is no chance of getting the job. Her perfect scenario ended the moment she woke up because once her perfect scenario had gone wrong, there was no plan B to follow – she didn't have something else she could wear, she didn't have alternative transport planned and she couldn't make up for her lateness by impressing with her knowledge of the job and the company. Her negative experience generates a huge drop in confidence and leaves her doubting her own ability to succeed in future projects.

Our second lady also knows her chances are high but not high enough to guarantee the job. She wants to do everything she can to improve her chances. She recognizes that the job could greatly improve her personal satisfaction by providing a bigger salary, more prospects and a potential to increase positive stimulation. By recognizing the incentive, she can decide on the level of commitment she is prepared to make. As the potential rewards are high, she has decided that getting this job will become her immediate priority. She knows she can increase her chances of getting the job by creating a good impression at the interview. To achieve this, she prepares a plan of action, so she can deal with potential problems before they occur and increase her knowledge of the situation.

Firstly she looks at what to wear. Will it need ironing or repairing or will she need a new outfit? Time needs to be set aside to do any of these. She also sets aside a back-up outfit, just in case. Then she looks at how to get to the interview. Her car has been playing up lately so does she get a cab, bus or put her car into the garage beforehand?

She has already decided to leave early and has found a coffee shop close by with good toilet facilities in case she needs a bit of a touch up. She has travelled the journey and found out exactly where she needs to go. Everything on her list goes through the same procedure of addressing the task, getting as much information as possible, then deciding on the most successful option and building in a back-up plan in case something unexpected happens.

She has researched the company, the job description and even tested her response to difficult questions. On the day of the interview, even if her car does break down or she snags her tights, she can still feel confident about getting through it all successfully because she will not be thrown when things don't go to plan. In fact, she will feel that it was even more of a success because she knows she could cope with the additional challenge.

The chances are, though, that the day will run smoothly because of her preparations. If, after all that, she doesn't get the job at least she can rationally learn from the experience because she knows there was nothing more she could have done. She will either decide that the position wasn't right for her anyway or she will know exactly what she needs to do to get a similar job. It hasn't limited her future chances or ability, if anything it will have improved them.

Preparation may seem boring but it can give you the opportunity to take a fantasy scenario and turn it into reality. In contrast, just hoping things will turn out okay is a recipe for disaster – and if you have a few negative experiences you will give up even trying.

Find Your Priority

The above scenario may seem very simplistic but it is not dissimilar to the types of situations we experience on a daily basis. A lot of living is this simplistic when you look at each incident in isolation. The reason our lives are complicated is because we usually have multiple situations happening all at once, leaving us with little time for the luxury of preparation. To deal with this, you need to decide which ones take priority and therefore require this kind of precise preparation. Preparation takes time but how much preparation is necessary depends on how great the reward, incentive and chances of success. You may feel that everything in your life is a priority but you may be wasting time on things that aren't that important because you feel that everything you do should be done to the same exacting high standard. With preparation, you will see what really is important and worth concentrating your efforts on. And if you can prioritize, your life will be less complicated – allowing you more time to enjoy living now.

Prepare To Work For Your Goal

I doubt there are many people who are reading this book out of desperation because they are unhappy with the outcome of a job interview – I imagine that the problems you have appear much worse. However, the principles of how you resolve them are still the same.

Look at your notes so far – have you ever considered taking the time to sit down and think practically about the issues you need to resolve? Probably not, because it isn't a particularly enjoyable experience – but to solve your problems you really need to get to grips with them.

Look at the earlier exercise and consider the following...

Can you relate to either of these women?
Do you always hope that things will turn out all right?
Do you always seem to be dealing with emergencies?
Can you never find the time to prepare?

Then ask yourself this ...

How important is making a change to you?
What do you need to consider before you attempt it?
What are your chances of success?
Can you improve your chances?
How?

Only by addressing these questions will you feel you have the ability and confidence to make a difference. First I would like you to try a little exercise just to get you to really focus on what your true priorities are, because these are the ones that will make your life happier and healthier.

Try This

Imagine you only have 48 hours left on this planet. Nothing awful is going to happen but some aliens have offered you a great opportunity in another galaxy and you couldn't resist. This means you have only 48 hours to see whoever you want, do whatever you want and say whatever you want. Fortunately your new alien friends have a galactic spaceship that can transport you anywhere in the world in no time, so you're not limited by travelling time. Your 48 hours is for you to live to the full.

This exercise is designed to make you realize what is really important in your life, what makes life worth living for you, what makes you happy, who you care about and where you feel happiest. Having done this exercise with many people, I can tell you that I have never heard anyone say, 'I wish I had spent more time in the office or arguing with my neighbour.'

I can also tell you that for most people, their plan is never very materialistic or ambitious. I find – and I include myself in this – that usually the time would be spent at a favourite beach or beauty spot, either on their own or with just one or two close family members or friends, with perhaps a larger party one evening. In fact, most people choose things that most of us could do on any weekend of the year. If something as simple as that is your ultimate pleasure, why are you not doing more of it?

If you are depriving yourself of these moments why is it a surprise that you are not happy? If you look at all the negative people and events that you would not count as an important aspect in your life, why are they dominating your life?

Of course, in reality, you do have responsibilities and commitments that take up the majority of your time – but do they really need to take over all of it?

Case History

I have had more than one client whose life has been made miserable by a family member, usually an in-law. They felt constantly criticized and humiliated, but obliged to spend a large amount of their own free time in the company of the abuser. When carrying out the above exercise, I set a deadline to prepare and prioritize. With the imposed restraint of a time scale, people are forced to focus and deal with their problem rather than denying and delaying it. Everyone goes through a thought process that involves looking at options and assessing and selecting those that have the best chance of a good result. For example, one lady decided to write a letter to the offending person but then felt this would take up too much of her precious time. She then decided to just call round and shout obscenities on the doorstep but concluded that it wasn't worth the emotional input. Eventually she decided not to bother doing anything as her time was too precious hence her 48 hours became problem-relative free. She had struck the offending relative out of her list of priorities very easily.

Making New Resolutions

Back in reality, with no deadline, it would not be necessarily advisable to do any of these things – but that is not the point of the exercise. What it demonstrates is how an unimportant issue can dominate to the detriment of what is really important. With a change in priority, this lady could begin to focus her emotional energy into important positive relationships, rather than wasting it on minor negative ones.

Not only did this exercise encourage her to experiment with a range of possible actions she hadn't considered before but it also set a deadline for her to resolve or come to terms with this unpleasant situation. Up until that point, she had been working on a small amount of fact and then filling in the gaps with a combination of assumption and personal insecurity. She was so bogged down with her own personal distress that her focus was always on the time spent with this unpleasant person. She had become completely oblivious to the fact that the majority of her time was spent elsewhere and that 99 per cent of the conversations she had were inoffensive.

By facing reality, she realized that it would be virtually impossible to change the offending person but she could change her own attitude and the level of importance she had bestowed on them. She was able to accept that if she wanted to be with the person she loved there would always be this negative aspect in the overall pleasurable package. For years her self-esteem had been undermined by this one peripheral person and she felt that her entire life was controlled by them. Doing the '48-hour' exercise made her realize that she had a whole array of options she could follow to regain control and that it was only her own attitude to the situation that was making it so intolerable.

She recognized that if her priority was to have a happy marriage then she needed to reduce the effects of this negative element and free up more time to enjoy the relationship she wanted to have with her husband. As she no longer saw this problem as important but more of a minor irritant in the grand scheme of things, she became more rational and objective about the situation, rather than seeing it as a direct personal attack. She now viewed her tormenter as an unhappy and lonely person whose insecurity had materialized into resentment. It wasn't a personal thing, anyone marrying her son would have had the same treatment. Instead of feeling dominated by this person, she now felt pity and this made a huge difference to the structure of the relationship. Of course, if she had concluded that her marriage was loveless, there would not have been much of an incentive to put up with either, so her plan would have been one of removing herself from the situation as painlessly as possible.

Your negative issues may be very different to this lady's but can you associate with her feelings of frustration and intimidation?

Is someone or something maintaining your negative situation?

Can you see it getting worse in the future?

Are you still holding out for a perfect solution?

You may have a different problem but the route to resolution is the same. Look at how you view your situation. A change in approach or attitude may not resolve it completely but it could make it much more manageable and tolerable. In her situation, the only real way to remove the problem was to also lose the thing she loved most of all. She took control and made a calculated compromise – and realistically this is the most likely way that you will achieve positive results in the long run.

What Did Your 48 Hours Say About You?

Look at what you wanted to do, where you wanted to be and who you wanted to be with. This is where your pleasure and satisfaction lie. If these things are not part of your life can you now see how important it is to reinstate them?

More time with those you love, more time with nature, more time to think and more time to consider your needs. That is what your body needs – not time spent with an aggressive boss or worrying about an irritating neighbour or the mother-in-law from hell.

If the things you wish for are impossible to bring back, then look at the positive emotion that they produced. This is what you really want to experience. You cannot always reinstate old loves, likes and needs. The old love may be gone forever and likes and needs from the past may no longer produce the positive responses they once did. What you are yearning for now is the positive emotion they brought and not necessarily the object that once created it. There are things in the future that could produce a similar response, or an even better one, but you do need to replace the ones you no longer have if you want to have a happy future.

Don't be despondent if you have no idea what to do in your 48 hours because nothing or nobody stands out as important or pleasurable. Finding happiness is not easy, which is why the pursuit of it can be such an uncertain and torturous route. You need to go through the pleasure and pain of experience and experiment to attain happiness so avoiding doing either will virtually guarantee an unhappy existence. You do need to gamble on something that has the potential to improve your life because you can never guarantee that it will. If you want to improve on your pleasure and satisfaction levels then preparation is the key. You need to experiment but you will want to do it without too many detrimental consequences and careful preparation enables you to do just that. Draw up a list of things you think would improve your life, make one a priority, get as much information as possible on it, prepare a strategy and set yourself a deadline to assess your progress.

Ask yourself ...

Could I make it work following this plan?

Do I want to make it work; will it be worth it?

If not, then go back to your list and try something else.

Dealing With Deadlines

Look at the questions asked so far in part two. Would your answers be different if you had to adhere to a deadline?

So far we have looked at how you can increase your chances of successfully changing your life. The final component of successful preparation is introducing a time scale to your plan. You know that if something has a tight timescale, it immediately becomes a priority. Your mind works like you do, with a 'jobs to do' list. It knows that it cannot sort everything out at once so it works on a priority system. The reason why so many of us do well in situations that have imposed deadlines – such as work – but have problems organizing time to enjoy life and achieve long-term ambitions is because life appears to have such a long timescale. You probably feel that you can get around to your dreams and goals another day, once you have sorted out the immediate problems of earning a living and getting the children off to school. However, that day never quite seems to become available. The longer you neglect your dreams and desires, the more the frustration, stress and resentment mounts up inside you. Eventually you'll reach breaking point, when either you can stand it no longer and walk away from everything or your body can stand it no longer and just starts to give up.

If you acknowledge a problem in its infancy, you can monitor and assess it in a rational way rather than in emotional or physical turmoil. You will then have time to research, work out a variety of options and then set a deadline to resolve or explore. For example, you can give a problem three months to see if it disappears on its own before you act, you can give yourself two weeks to gain a greater understanding of the situation before you attempt to deal with it or you can ask someone else to help but assess your combined progress in a month. Setting a series of deadlines as you progress will help you prevent the problem reappearing and ensure that no other problems build up in the process.

It is unlikely that you will reach your deadline and find that everything has gone to plan, on time and produced a perfect result. What a deadline will do is give you an opportunity to assess and review your progress to see if you are moving in the right direction.

Working to a timescale will not only encourage you to act but will help you discover if your actions are working and if not, why not. You can learn new techniques that will speed the process up and you can decide at an early stage whether you really want to do it anyway. Changing anything in your life will involve action. Preparing to change will make it easier to act and setting a timescale will make that action more effective. So what are you waiting for? Stop putting things off and prepare to change your life for the better.

Summary

- Recognize Your True Incentive – what is going to keep you motivated?
- Prepare For A Greater Reward – how are you going to make it work?
- Don't Be Afraid To Experiment – are you limiting your outlook?
- Learn From Past Disappointments – what can help you now that you didn't know then?
- Set A Time Scale For Success – how long will this realistically take you?

Embrace Reality

When you have problems, reality is something you may find hard to face, but what if your problems had been created, repeated or were being maintained by an inability to see things as they really are?

You could benefit from reassessing your view of reality if you...

- Often use the phrases 'if only', 'should have been' and 'why me' in conversation.
- Have been in a situation where those around you could see a potential problem arising long before you would accept it could occur.
- Get angry about, or disregard, advice, concerns or a warning from a close friend or family member.

- Feel that negative aspects of your life have become impossible to change.
- Are not satisfied unless everything is perfect.

It is difficult to define reality because it is so different for all of us. A lot of what you see may be what you would like to see or is based purely on an accumulation of assumptions and is not a true picture of what is really going on. Of course we would all like to have perfect relationships, careers, children, health and lifestyles but perfection is virtually impossible to maintain so we often focus on the perfect as our benchmark and hope that we will progress towards it. These are your dreams for the future and it is the expectation of these that will bring you a large part of the pleasure and satisfaction you need to make life worthwhile. If you are always making progress to narrow the gap between your present reality and your future dream, then you should be content with life – even if you never actually reach that perfect state.

Conversely, you will experience unhappiness and dissatisfaction if that gap starts to widen. However, these negative responses are there to help you act on the imbalance and get you back on track. Problems can occur when you continually refuse to accept that the gap is getting wider and you are further away from achieving a need or desire. If you are living your life on expectation, simply hoping things will improve rather than working to resolve the negative state that you are in, then every day will be a constant source of disappointment. The difficulties you have will appear impossible to resolve because you can only change what really exists, not a fantasy reality that you have cooked up in your head.

If you have been unable to change aspects of your life, even though you know they are making you unhappy or unhealthy, you need to ensure that you are starting from a realistic standpoint and that your future expectations are achievable, otherwise it will be hard to make or maintain any change at all.

To be able to make progress, you need to have a starting point, therefore understanding what is really happening *now* will make it easier for you to see what you can realistically change to build a better future.
If you ...

- Regularly get angry and frustrated during day-to-day routine tasks like taking the children to school or driving to work.
- Feel that people are repeatedly letting you down.
- Find that the only way you can get anyone to help you is to nag or shout.
- Feel that you should have achieved so much more with your life.
- Suffer from severe jealousy or envy.
- Walk down the street and think that everyone looks so much better, happier, slimmer, brighter or healthier than you.

... then you need to address your view of reality.

Choose Reality

Imagine you have to drive to work each day through the city centre in the rush hour. What is your attitude towards the journey?

Would you hate it?

Is this because there would be loads of traffic, with the roads full of people cutting you up and doing stupid things? If so, then what you're probably annoyed about is the fact that without all the traffic, you could easily do the journey in a quarter of the time without all the aggravation. If this was your attitude then it's likely that you will regularly arrive late and angry and greet all your work colleagues with a full rundown on all the idiots who made this particular journey a bad one.

This daily event may be your reality but it is not 'factual'. What you would be doing is trying to live in some self-created fantasy land. There is a chance that you could do the journey quickly, find absolutely no traffic on the road and not get caught for speeding – but it's not very likely. A realistic journey to work at that time of day would be one that involved lots of traffic, frayed tempers and lots of people driving badly – because most of the people on that road would be living in the same little unreality bubble as you.

If you accepted the facts of reality then you could do something about it. You could avoid the negative elements of the situation by leaving earlier, or you could change your job, hours, mode of transport or simply accept that the journey will be long and unpleasant. If you were to choose the latter, you could find ways to improve on the journey by making it the time to listen to music, learn a new language or even time to practice some new relaxation techniques. The point is you now have choices and once you recognize this you can start to take control. Once you have accepted the reality, the task now becomes something you are doing because you choose to do it, not because you are forced to. You do that journey because you need to get to work. You need to get to work because you like the money or the social interaction or the sense of achievement. Whichever one it is, you are doing it for your own personal satisfaction. If you are not, you know you have to do something else.

When you choose to do something it is because you feel it is beneficial to you, therefore the chances are that you won't feel so grumpy when you arrive to work and you will usually be able to arrive on time because you will have made the time to get there. If you do have a better than usual journey to work, even if it was just because nobody cut you up, you will arrive even happier. Your overall change in attitude will improve your relationship with your work colleagues and could improve your chances of success because your boss will see you as someone who is punctual, bright and copes well with difficult situations.

Spatial Perception

One of the most wonderfully logical processes the brain uses is spatial perception. Every time you make a physical request of the body, for example to enable you to walk across a room or pick up a glass, the brain has to decide what the body needs to do to make this action occur in the easiest possible way. It calculates the distance, potential obstacles and scale of urgency, and weighs up the amount of resources and depth of ability it has available to it. Emotional requests are subject to the same process. The brain needs to calculate the 'distance' to determine how long it will realistically take to achieve your demands – bearing in mind any existing obstacles such as anyone or anything likely to hold you back – and take account of the sense of urgency, calculated from how much longer you can tolerate your current situation. It then combines this information with your emotional and physical state and your depth of knowledge to see if what is being requested is feasible. This calculation will establish whether the task is possible and, if it is, how long it will take and what result can be realistically expected. The level of success is measured by how much the reality of the result meets with your expectation.

$$\text{TASK} = \frac{(\text{DISTANCE} + \text{OBSTACLES} + \text{URGENCY})}{(\text{RESOURCES} + \text{ABILITY})} = \text{RESULT}$$

If your resources and ability are adequate enough to deal easily with the distance, obstacles and urgency, the result will be good; if they are inadequate, the results are likely to be disappointing.

For example, often you cannot do something for the simple reason that your body does not have enough energy. Imagine you wanted to do a simple task like walk across the room but your body lacks the energy to move – you are going to feel pretty fed-up about it but, unfortunately, that is the reality of the situation. Although the reality is not as you would have hoped, by confronting it you can take steps to deal with and improve on your situation, rather than being defeated by it. In this situation you would need to address why your energy is so low and combine this information with positive steps to restore it, which should soon have you successfully walking across the room again. Even if you could not fully explain why you had such low energy, accepting that you did would enable you to work with your body to find a solution that would help you in future.

If you do not accept the reality of the situation and refuse to believe that your body is incapable of crossing the room because 'it's easy, everyone does it and I had no trouble yesterday', not only are you exhausting your body further by forcing it to continue trying but you are also making the problem impossible to resolve because you are refusing to accept that there is a problem. If you persist in trying to make your body do something that it is incapable of you can create a much bigger health problem – denying a problem exists can often become more damaging than the initial problem itself.

Assess Your Current Position

In order for spatial perception to work, the body must be aware of its exact position. The brain cannot calculate how to get somewhere until it has established its existing position and assessed the situation. Basically it has to know where you are now before it can make a decision on how to help you get to where you want to go next. If you wanted to pick up a glass for example, and your brain had no idea how far the relevant limb was from not just the glass but other items in the surrounding area, it would not be able to calculate how far or in which direction it would need to move your limb to produce a successful result, hence it wouldn't even try. Not only does the brain have to coordinate the movements of the body but, before it acts, it also has to assess the potential effect of the intended action on the surrounding environment – this prevents it creating a new problem in the process of resolving an existing one. To do all this, your brain needs to deal with the reality of the here and now so that it can feel confident that future actions will produce a favourable result. If your brain feels uncertain, it will prevent your body from acting and feelings of fear will arise.

To enable things to occur, the body needs to go through a process of comparing desires with actual ability. If your desires are way above your capabilities, then your body will not act on your instruction because it knows it will not be able to achieve what you want. If you recognize that your desires are way beyond your immediate capabilities then your body will encourage you to reach an achievable compromise or help you to improve your abilities so that you will be capable of realizing your desires in the future. This is how the body likes to operate – by using rational thought processes to implement beneficial physical responses.

Five reasons why your body might be stopping you:

1 Because your expectations are too high.
2 Because it fears for your safety.
3 Because its capabilities are too low.
4 Because it needs more information.
5 Because it does not have enough sustainable energy.

These are the issues that need to be addressed if you want your body to respond to your demands.

The brain makes decisions about what to do based on the information that results from your emotional needs, environment and capabilities. Unfortunately this information can be based on a small collection of facts and a large amount of assumption to fill in the gaps. This is why we so readily put two and two together to make eight.

Making Assumptions

Your brain contains so much stored information that on a day-to-day basis it would be impossible to sift through it all in order to make a decision. You therefore have to make judgements about what is likely to happen based on previous experience and anecdotal evidence. As humans are not isolated in their experience, your brain will register 'most likely' outcomes from society as a whole and the experience of other people to try and improve your chances of making better decisions about your future.

Each day you have to make a multitude of decisions, which leaves you with little time to assess all the available information. As a result, each decision you make will be based on assumptions formed from what you already know. I am sure you have experienced strange occurrences like seeing someone when there is no one there or knowing who is calling you before you pick up the phone. We all get excited about spooky coincidences but a great many of them occur because your brain has been presented with a few prominent facts and has immediately filled in the missing gaps with information in its memory bank.

Your brain can jump to a conclusion with only a small amount of fact available to it, so, for example, it can assume that the person most likely to phone you is someone you talk to a lot or someone you haven't heard from for a while. It may appear strange if you had just thought about that person prior to them ringing, but that is only because they happen to be in your immediate memory. Coincidences do occur so although the chances of the person you are thinking about actually phoning you at that point may be slim, they were probably thinking exactly the same as you – that you hadn't spoken to each other for a while and hence they picked up the phone. You do not register when, as is more usual, it is not a coincidence, because no connection can be made.

Your brain will jump to a conclusion if a coincidence has triggered off a memory reaction. Your brain may need more information to make a rational decision but if, for instance, you are desperate to see someone or achieve something then it will respond to the slightest similarity.

The brain has to analyse everything that you come into contact with to see if it bears a resemblance to your desire. It then fills in the missing pieces from past experience. This is why you might see things that are not there or things that you would like to see, rather than what is really there – because you have an ideal image in your head. If you do not give your brain new information or long for things from your past that are no longer achievable then your image of reality can become distorted or irrational.

An Example

If you see a strange man running towards you, you could assume he was about to harm you. Even though this may never have happened to you before, you will be aware that it has happened to others and therefore could happen to you. This generates feelings of anxiety and distress and your brain registers a connection between men running and distress. Now, every time you encounter a similar scenario, you could experience a negative anxious response, even though the anxiety is not necessary or rational. Your first thought is that this person is a potential source of harm and you fail to consider all the non-threatening reasons why a man may be running in your direction – for example to catch a bus, to hand you back something you have dropped and so on.

Unfortunately, in such situations, it is all too easy to remember the negative and discount the positive or mundane – after all, shocking or unusual events are widely reported but the millions of non-threatening or pleasant events that occur daily are never reported because they are the norm. In this situation, you will find it hard to realistically assess the true likelihood of harm occurring because you are not considering all the information required to make a balanced decision.

Look at how this example relates to you.

Do you repeatedly experience the same negative responses?

Do you panic in new or non-threatening environments?

What is it you fear?

Do you assume the worst in every situation?

Do you always attempt to resolve things in the same way?

Does this negativity limit your life?

It would help you to keep a diary to see if a pattern emerges. List all the things you associate with your problem. You need to find out if it is the cause or just a trigger for negative emotions. To be effective your treatment should deal with the cause, therefore locating the true facts behind your current situation will provide an important stepping-stone to resolution.

Learn To Accept Your Reality

You have probably gathered by now that life can be hard going sometimes. Those tough times are made easier by the pleasure and satisfaction in our lives. For this reason, it is commonplace for people to cling to the last remnants of something good, rather than acknowledge that the pleasure has gone. It may be hard to face the fact that a once seemingly perfect situation no longer exists, or a desired one is currently unachievable, but the only way you can begin to improve is through accepting the reality of your current situation.

We all have people or places that remind us of happy times and every time we think of them or visit them, we feel a positive emotion. While that person or place is supplying us with positive emotion, we remain happy with the situation. However, if your desire is to experience a positive emotion from someone that makes you unhappy, or if you still want to feel the positive emotions you once felt from something that now brings dissatisfaction, this could be a sign that a gap has appeared between reality and your desire to maintain or create a dream. Similarly, if you once felt full of energy and now feel tired all the time your desire will be to regain your once high energy levels. If you wake up every morning disappointed that you are still tired and spend the day being angry about your inability to do things then by the end of the day you will be even more exhausted and miserable. If you accept that your body is tired and needs to rest, you will attempt to help it rather than resent it. When problems start to emerge it can be easier to refuse to accept they exist because you prefer to hold onto the dream of how things were or should be. Unfortunately, this can bring greater anxiety, as people often convince themselves that the problem is a result of their own inadequacies – or something loosely associated with the problem – rather than believe their beloved place, person, lifestyle or whatever could have any faults at all.

Emotion By Association

People's emotional reactions are a very subjective thing because everyone has different wishes, desires and experiences. It is so easy to forget this and fall into the trap of assuming that because you like something everyone else will too. For example, I have one particular favourite place and love anywhere or anything that reminds me of it. However, I have a friend who had a terrible accident at the same place and, not surprisingly, she hates it because it brings back very unhappy emotions. Not only that, she dislikes going anywhere that has similar scenery, even though she loved that type of landscape before the incident. I call this 'emotion by association' because it is an emotional reaction to something that bears only a coincidental relationship to the cause of the original emotional experience.

This type of association can result in a repeated reaction occurring because the brain is being supplied with emotional information that is not necessarily relevant.

List as many different emotions as you can think of: happiness, sadness, fear, enthusiasm, elation etc.

What do you immediately think of with each emotion?

Is it a colour, person, place, event; what is it?

Is there a justifiable reason for that association?

Can this association positively improve your life as it is today?

If it does not then now is the time to change that association.

Memory Training

As soon as you are born, you begin filling up your memory banks. Your brain has two types of memory, short and long term. Short-term memory deals with day-to-day stuff such as who you are, where you live, who you live with, where the shops are and what you were talking about five minutes ago. Long-term memory works on a need-to-know basis.

The brain is like a giant computer with the capacity to store every sight, sound and sensation you come into contact with. It feels, quite rightly, that too much information would only confuse you. For example, if you set your brain the task of getting you to work in the morning it would not be of any value to you at that time to know that the supermarket you just passed is doing a buy-one-get-one-free offer on all boxes of chocolate and the lady at the bus stop is wearing a really neat pair of suede boots. You just need to know what is happening around you that could affect your journey to work. Only when you realize later that Mother's Day is fast approaching and you also have a desperate need to buy shoes does the information on the chocolate and boots surface from nowhere. Suddenly you know exactly where to buy chocolates and what style of footwear you are looking for. It is the job of your brain to weed out the bits it feels have any relevance to your here and now and store the rest away for future use. Only when you change your priorities, will new information become apparent. We often talk about fate and things appearing at the right time but often those opportunities have always been there, they have only become apparent because a change in priority or perspective has made seemingly non-important stored information suddenly relevant.

Your memory needs retraining if ...

It has only one solution to a problem and this never works.

You repeatedly make the same mistakes.

You feel constantly frustrated with your efforts.

You never see problems until it is too late to avoid them.

Your life seems to be an endless round of setbacks.

You can retrain your memory by ...

Concentrating your energies on what you can do rather than what you cannot – small positive steps forward will make a big difference over time.

Giving yourself time to think through a problem and draw up a list of things that will help – drawing up a plan will keep you in control.

Finding out how other people work through their problems – you will certainly find some original new solutions to try.

Making a decision to end the cycle – look at the negative pattern you are in and take steps to break it.

Focusing on looking for solutions rather than dwelling on the problem – keep your mind open to what is going on around you. The more you know, the easier it will be to deal with the reality.

Never Stop Learning

If a new situation occurs, then your mind will trawl through its database to see if there is anything relevant that could help. This is why it is important to keep learning new skills and increasing your knowledge. The better informed you are, the greater your ability to cope and therefore the more favourable the result. It also explains why the same situation can be a nightmare for one person and thrilling for another. By increasing knowledge, personal experience and your ability to cope you can have more realistic expectations, greater skills and more confidence and security, and this means that there is the potential to turn a nightmare task into something more acceptable.

Very few of us would want to walk into a burning building, for example, but a fireman does just that on a regular basis. That is because he knows everything there is to know about fire, has practiced going into burning buildings many times and has the equipment to do so. The danger is still there but his fear of it has diminished to an extent that enables him to succeed in a task that most would never consider undertaking.

The brain applies the same combination of learning and experience to recurring situations by accessing its 'file' on how you dealt with similar past situations. This is known as memory training and it's obviously very useful because it means you can use existing skills to deal with familiar situations. In theory, this should mean that you can deal quickly and successfully with recurrent problems. Unfortunately, there is a downside because the brain will programme in how you first solved the problem and not whether this was the most effective or efficient way of solving it. Unless you take steps to improve, your brain will rely entirely on these old familiar patterns – even if the result was not all it could be. For example, if you buy a new video but try to set it up without the instruction manual, you will eventually work out a system for use but it may involve wasted hours trying to get it to work in the same way the old one did, or only using a certain brand of video tape because it always used to work best. Of course if you gained more knowledge about the video by reading the manual or asking an expert, the chances are you would find a much faster and more effective way of using your video, which would mean a lot less strain on you and the machine. It would also give you more confidence in your abilities, a simpler life and a healthier attitude because you would be more in touch with the facts rather than simply hoping for the best.

If you do not continue learning and rely only on your existing skills, you will find that you're more likely to use the same limited coping techniques over and over again. In fact it is often the way you deal with a problem that makes it recur, because you repeat the same mistakes over and over again rather than looking for a way to solve it once and for all. The memory will only provide the information demanded of it, which is why, for instance, someone can answer obscure questions in a pub quiz but can't seem to stop themselves having repeated relationships with the same type of emotionally draining no-hoper.

If you are repeatedly not coming up with the right answers then ask yourself what your memory needs ...

Does it need new information?

Am I asking it the right questions?

Long-standing problems can often be resolved if you just change your perspective.

An Example

Think about how a young child attracts attention. It has limited means of communication but has to rely on others for its survival. If crying gets attention then it will continue to use crying as a means of attracting attention until it learns that there are different ways of getting what it wants. It will use crying if it is hungry or uncomfortable but laughing and smiling if it wants love and affection. As the child grows and acquires new skills, it will learn that crying isn't as effective as asking politely for what it wants and that being pleasant results in more positive attention. If that child continues to rely on the crying-equals-attention technique it will grow up using the same negative emotions to get the things it wants. This is not only unpleasant for the child but also for those around it. They could also grow to become demanding and abusive, which means that it will be harder for them to get help and form positive, lasting relationships. This of course will only generate more frustration and increase their aggression and agitation. If they do not learn to break the cycle of repeating this ineffective technique, they will continue using it into adulthood, thereby increasing their emotional instability.

Knowledge Is Power

Think of how you communicate with others – do you use negative responses to get attention or to get things done?

If you use negative responses repeatedly, you will be in danger of depriving yourselves of the positive stimuli you need to keep you happy. You need to experience positive feedback to maintain a healthy level of happiness, therefore if you constantly rely on negative responses it will be difficult to experience any positive stimulation. Even though you may well be aware that these negative responses produce unsatisfactory results, you may still feel afraid to try anything different because you fear that you could make things worse or get no response at all. The scary thing about changing a negative habit is the fear of not knowing what will happen if you stop and not knowing what you will replace it with.

If you don't know how to improve things in your life then you need more information. Knowledge is empowering. The more you know about something, the less you need to rely on guesswork and assumption. The more facts you have at your disposal, the more rational you can be in your thought processes. And the more you understand reality, the better your chances of a beneficial result. If you need answers, you have to start asking questions and the questions in this book are designed to help you with that process of discovery.

It's time to find out what your fear factor is. What don't you know about your situation?

Accept Or Change

If you want to change your life then choices have to be made. In theory, you have already taken the first step by wanting to change – but you need to actively choose between accepting the situation as it is or changing it. If you are hoping for the best of both worlds and not achieving it, one solution could be to accept one element as negative to get the positive benefit from the other. Alternatively, you could change your situation or your attitude towards it.

Look at the three options available:

1 Stay as you are – can you stay as you are; is there any chance of future happiness?

If the answer is no then ...

2 Accept that there is a conflict with your desires. Accept what is negative and concentrate on the things that will bring positive results. Can you accept that some desires in your life are preventing you from achieving others?

If you cannot do this then ...

3 Change – look for new sources of pleasure and satisfaction. Can you improve some aspects of your life, even if they appear unrelated to your problem, to make the problem less dominant in your life?

Open Your Mind To Suggestions

Think back to how the brain filters out information. You tell it what is important, what your priority is and it will relay information back it feels is relevant to that issue. If a particular annoyance starts to dominate your life then the brain will continually supply you with information that relates to your problem – hence virtually everything you see and do will seem in some way connected with that one problematic thing. For example, if you go on a diet and decide to give up chocolate, you will see slim people everywhere and it will appear that every shop sells chocolate. The reality is that only a small percentage of people are slim and no, chocolate is not a compulsory item in all shops. A world full of slim people and chocolate has become your reality because that is the only information you appear interested in. If you have an issue that you cannot resolve, it appears that the whole world is full of people who are free from that issue. You imagine everyone else is full of energy, happy, with partners, has well-behaved children, is rich and successful and so on. If you focus continually on one negative issue, your brain will supply you with an endless stream of information relating to that topic. If you have no energy, then your brain will bring your attention to anyone who looks lively because they have what you want.

When I was ill, I initially refused to accept the extent of my ill health. I hated resting and if I felt the slightest improvement I was out trying to take over the world again. This meant that I never really rested because I was anxious and dissatisfied when I couldn't get out of bed and physically exhausted myself when I could. The turning point came when I accepted that I was ill and the only thing I was capable of doing successfully was resting. I changed my whole attitude to rest. I saw it as a positive thing, something that would help my body recover and, because of that, I tried to introduce other positive changes into my life to aid my recovery, such as relaxation techniques and things that I could do that brought me pleasure.

My mind had been focused on this one overwhelming problem and everything I did was associated with it. I imagined everyone I saw was fit and healthy and everyone I spoke to was achieving something wonderful. I was still living in a world that was exciting and happy but I was the one thing in it that was a disappointment. Unpleasant as it was, accepting my reality gave me a range of options. I could stay as I was and learn to accept it or try to change by improving my knowledge of the situation and experimenting with new ideas. Whatever I decided to do, it meant that I could have control over what I was doing and could decide what did and didn't work for me.

This is how I started to address my reality. I looked at my three options and came up with the following questions and answers:

- Do I want to stay as I am?
  No
- Do I accept my situation?
  No, I need to change it.
- Can I change it?
  No because I'm too tired and don't understand why I am so ill.
- Why am I so tired?
  I do not know why I'm ill but I do know that I am tired because I will not accept my situation and this is making me anxious, unhappy and exhausted.
- If I accept that I am tired and unhappy can I find constructive ways to improve my situation?
  The answer to this was my turning point because in answering yes, I could finally act positively and do something – even if that something seemed quite minor and unrelated.

When it comes to health and well-being, everything is connected because nothing in the body works in isolation. It was these early, small steps that led to a greater understanding of my condition and, eventually, my recovery. I was unhappy because I felt so ill, but I allowed that unhappiness with my illness to spill over into areas of my life that should still have been a source of happiness. This then made me unhappy with all of my life, which of course meant I felt even more physically exhausted, and so the vicious circle continued. Once I took positive steps – no matter how small – to improve my physical state, my mental state also improved because it enabled me to see my illness as a part of my life and not the whole. At the time I could not make a big difference to my physical state but I could concentrate on other aspects in my life that could potentially relieve me of some of the distress, rather than abandoning them because of my ill health.

Now look again at your options; do you want to stay as you are? If the answer is no, then look at positive small steps you can realistically make now.

- List your options – what can you do now that will make your life more bearable?
- Get more information and concentrate on things that work.
- Look at the positive and negative elements in your life – are the negative ones overshadowing the positive? If they are, put more time and energy into those positive elements.
- Trust your instincts. If you are confident with your choice, then you should feel excited and not frightened. If you feel afraid, then something is still not right and you need to start the process again.

Small Steps Reap Big Results

When I was ill, my life was pretty unpleasant but by compartmentalizing and examining all the components of my life, I could see that I had been failing to recognize the positive steps available to me because I had become dominated by the negative. It was a case of stripping back and rebuilding. My recovery started when I concentrated my energies into the positive elements of my life and began to look for new ones. This helped me to look to the future. The goal of getting better became my priority. I recognized that, as with any task, there would be effort involved so I would need to plan, organize and take control of my own health. Once I introduced new positive things into my life, these became my focus and this helped me to accept or change the negative.

So many of my clients begin by saying, 'Everything in my life is awful', when, in fact, only one or two things are really awful. Unfortunately, over time a few negative factors can begin to override all the positive aspects of life until everything really does become awful. It is important, therefore, that you separate the negative from the positive and what you can still potentially achieve.

Look For The Cause

Many of the negative symptoms we experience are the result of an underlying problem. Your body is a series of interconnecting systems and any one cause can generate a multitude of diverse symptoms as the effects ripple out. Negative symptoms such as pain, fatigue, weight problems and unhappiness are there to tell us that there is a problem; they are not the problem in themselves. If you treat symptoms as the problem you will never address the underlying cause and your success will be limited. However, if you treat them as a guide, they can lead you to where the real problem lies.

Sometimes your body will deliberately suppress the reality of a situation as part of the recovery process. If you experience a major trauma such as bereavement, you will go through a series of emotions that will allow the body and mind to adapt to your new circumstances. There is a recognized set pattern of emotions that the body undergoes following a trauma. This process includes denial and numbness, because the body believes that too much reality all at once could be devastating. At some point in our lives we all feel that we have been blind not to see the reality of a situation earlier but often the body feels that slow realization is the healthier option. It is easy, in hindsight, to persecute yourself for not realizing something sooner but the chances are that if you had been fully aware, you may not have been able to deal emotionally with the magnitude of the problem.

In such circumstances, a more likely cause of stress to the body is becoming stuck in a negative emotion, such as anger or guilt, as you attempt to sort out your problems. The body is designed to deal with passing emotional phases without incurring too much harm. In fact, the idea is that you learn and improve as a result of the experience. However, a prolonged period of negative emotion or worst still, never moving on from it at all, will result in both mental and physical damage.

The Flaws Of Perfection

Dwelling on why things are never perfect and blaming it on external situations will not help you improve a situation.

You know you have a problem with perfection when ...

- You have too many things that must be done every day.
- You get frustrated with the way other people do things, or don't.
- You expect to get praise and recognition from others.

- You hate things upsetting your routine.
- You often wonder why you bother.

If makes no difference if the upset or harm caused is intentional or not, the damage and method of recovery can still be the same. If someone ran over your foot in a car for example, it wouldn't make any difference to the injury if it was deliberate or an accident and the method of repairing it would be the same. Emotionally, you wouldn't feel that different either. You would still feel a sense of anger and vulnerability, they would simply be at different intensities.

The body has a set routine for recovery and you need to work with it to reach a successful conclusion. The body accepts that what has happened has happened and it can do nothing to change that fact. All it can concentrate on is making the best of the future from what it has available in the present – and this is what you need to do if you want to move to a more positive existence. If things have gone wrong then be prepared to sulk, cry or grieve – whatever you feel, accept it as part of the recovery process. In the short term it helps, but if you want to achieve a happier and healthier state you need to keep moving forward by concentrating on a better future.

Remember ...

- You can never change the past, you can only use your past experience to influence your future.
- Negative symptoms are there for a reason, dealing with that reason will set you on the road to recovery.
- Your body only wants to do what is best for you, so listen to what it is telling you.
- If you are stuck in a negative emotional pattern, it's time to move on.
- All your negative responses will be interlinked; if you cannot deal with one, concentrate on another.

Case History

A lady in her late 40s came to me complaining of years of fatigue and other stress-related problems such as muscular pain and backache. The first thing I noticed about her was that she was carrying a very large and very old handbag. I commented on this and she proudly told me that it was a treasured 18th birthday present. To me it represented a sentence of 30 years poor posture, which was evident in the fact that she had one shoulder visibly higher and rounder than the other. Although this may seem a small thing, any prolonged negative stress on the body – whether physical or mental – can only have a detrimental effect on its health and well-being. The effect of the bag on its own was not enough to generate the problems she was experiencing but if you added it to all the other negative elements in her life over the years, it was another contributory factor in the general overload her body was experiencing.

Not only was this handbag a physical drain on the body, it had even become a part of her emotional baggage. She associated the bag with happier times and clung on to it rather than recreate that happiness in the here and now. When I suggested she got a new and smaller bag she became very defensive and refused to listen to any reasons why she might benefit from a change.

It is important to recognize that it is not the size of the issue that is important – it is how you deal with it. If your physical and mental resources are constantly being used to deal with a combination of small but on-going stressful situations that affect your health and well-being, then your ability to cope with unexpected or major incidents will be dramatically reduced.

People often tell me that things only started to go wrong for them after a mentally-draining event – such as a bereavement, the birth of a child etc. – or as a result of an illness or accident. However, these things are only the trigger. Your body is designed to deal with traumatic physical and mental one-offs. Life will always hand these out, particularly when you least expect them. What is most likely to cause your body damage is the combination of negative elements and habits you pick up and add on through life. These slowly drain your resources and make it harder for your body to cope with the uncertainties that life throws at you.

Before my illness got so bad that it forced me to stop and sort myself out, I had had years of ill health – endless viruses and infections, suspected mumps, glandular fever ... I also had a huge amount of stress from work, a failing relationship and family problems, so I never had time to stop and rest, sleep properly, enjoy a holiday or follow a balanced diet. But I did make sure I swam a mile a day, even if I didn't get to the pool until midnight! Oh, and I liked to party until dawn. When I back-track and lay it out like this it's obvious why I ended up washed up and burnt out for four years. If I had addressed the lesser issues earlier and stopped them building up, I would never have got to that stage.

Take A Positive Step Forwards

Do you remember how your stress response likes to operate? It likes an incentive, followed by decision, action, a result and an assessment. Your brain follows the same procedure of events.

Organize Your Efforts

Anything you take on, even if it is designed to provide pleasure or satisfaction, will involve some sort of effort. This necessitates using your bodily resources and, even if you are super fit, there will still be a limit to the amount of energy your body can produce in one go. When the body has a lot to deal with, it will attempt to prioritize. However, if you insist that everything is equally demanding, it is left with no option but to distribute the resources evenly. This will mean that the more demands you

The Route To Success

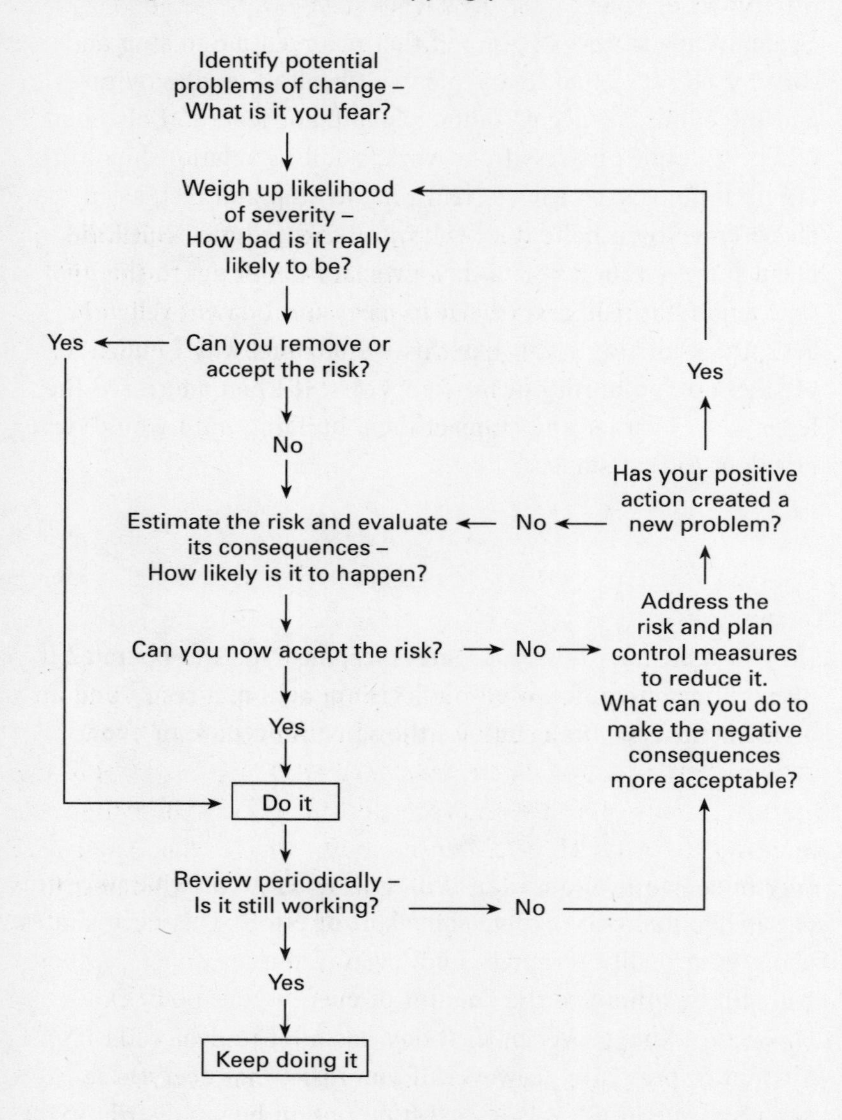

have, the more thinly your resources will be spread. This can lead to half-hearted or ineffectual attempts that could fizzle out long before any satisfactory result is achieved. If your body feels that the resources available are very low, it won't even attempt what you are asking of it. This leads to frustration and disappointment because the mind is willing but the body says no.

Try This

The following exercise can help you make a quick decision about what can be done now, what can safely be set aside till later and what really is and isn't important. It was originally designed as a time management tool so it really is a quick way of assessing your priorities.

The Four Ds

Do it
Delay it
Delegate it
or Dump it

Write down all the tasks you need to do or want to do then divide them into one of the four groups shown above – you have no other choices. For example, when the post arrives in the morning, glance through it and decide what you can deal with immediately, what needs closer attention, what can be handed over to someone else to deal with and what is of no interest to you at all.

Do It Now

These are your priority jobs.

If it's a small job, such as signing a form, or an annoying or urgent one that an immediate phone call can resolve, then do it straight away. If you do this you have immediately reduced your workload and also stopped yourself from becoming too anxious or upset by dwelling on something unpleasant. Don't give yourself time to dwell on or over-exaggerate a problem if you can address it immediately. Unexpected and unpleasant things can quite literally land on your doorstep but most of the anxiety they generate is as a result of not fully understanding their potential consequences because you do not, at this stage, have a full understanding of the problem or any control over it. By doing something constructive immediately you can occupy your mind with the practicality of resolution. Using your time now to gather facts means you will quickly be aware of what needs to be done, rather than leaving your mind to wander through a fantastical world of fearful assumptions.

Delay It

These are the things that need to be done but cannot be dealt with immediately.

You could be delaying something because you don't understand it fully and would like time to gather more information before making a decision on it, or it could simply be a task that doesn't need to be sorted out until later. There is a thin line between choosing to delay something and just ignoring it. You need to be organized about delaying things, so anything you set aside to be dealt with in the future should be classed as an ongoing project not something that you will 'get round to at some point'. Most things can't be resolved in one hit but you can do a bit now, then plan a time in the future to do a bit more. If it is something that doesn't need to be done now you still need to allocate time later to do something about it – otherwise you will either forget to do it and cause more problems or you'll be constantly reminding yourself not to forget to do it.

Even if you need or want to delay a task, you can still be working on preparation to help you resolve it later. You cannot and do not need to do everything now but often if you neglect something you feel you have failed at it. Giving yourself time to deal with things over a structured period can prevent mistakes occurring as a result of rushing in unprepared. It also removes the disappointment that arises from feeling you have given up something you always wanted to do because you haven't got time to do it immediately.

Delegate It

If you have reached this point in the exercise then all your priorities should have been recognized and taken care of. Whatever remains, you can now get rid of without it involving too much time and effort, after all if it hasn't been dealt with by now it cannot be important. You either need to let someone else deal with it or just decide it is not worth bothering with. Many of us, it appears, have a problem with delegation. I, like everyone else I'm sure, know exactly how I like something done, do it better than anyone else and in the shortest possible time. It's a fair comment because we all work from different agendas and for different incentives therefore it's obvious that we would do something well if the result had a direct influence on us. If somebody else did the same job for you, they would have less of an incentive to get things right because, at the end of the day, it would have little impact on them. You either need to accept that not everything needs to be done perfectly or inspire others to have the same strong incentive so they will want to do it as well you do.

Dump It

It should now be clear where your real priorities lie. Anything that you've classified in the 'dump it' category is obviously of no relevance or importance to you and can just be disposed of. By now you should already have a pile of more interesting, essential or demanding things to do that need your time and energy. If you have a problem de-cluttering, remind yourself what is the worst thing that can happen if you get rid of it. As yet I have never been struck down by lightning for chucking out that impulse-buy that was the latest fashion but looks awful on me, or had the heavy mob arrive on my doorstep when I didn't return some catalogue prize draw guarantee form.

I knew someone who kept the tail of a pet mouse for over 30 years. They were really upset when it died and they kept the tail to remind them of how upset they had been. One tail on its own is not a major collection but if you keep a memento of every emotional incident in your life then it soon starts to stack up. If you store too many things from your past there will never be any room to bring in new things. I'm not just talking about cluttering your life up with physical objects, but also the great weight of emotional baggage that goes with them. You need things to remind you of the past so that you can review and assess your progress and remember the things that have made a difference to your life. Memories can provide comfort but you need a sense of proportion. Cherish and learn from memories and mementos that are important or relevant and dispose of the ones that are not. Crying over a dead mouse at five years old shouldn't really be of any relevance 30 years on.

Categorizing things according to the '4Ds' is a very useful mental exercise but it also provides a useful analogy with how your physical body likes to operate. The body is keen to act as soon as a problem appears and therefore a great deal of anxiety and stress can be caused by not tackling problems immediately. By using this exercise you can make progress quickly on the essential things, like restoring health for example, while other problems like secondary relationship issues or future career ambitions can be put on the back burner until you feel ready to deal with them. Once your health improves and you have time to deal with your relationship problems or assess your career, it may already seem easier to resolve because you will be feeling happier in your self and less emotionally sensitive. Indeed, you may not even need to deal with it as you may well realize that it was not important – you had simply viewed it as a problem because of your attitude at the time.

Things in your life that you can '4D' ...
Friends
Family
Health
Emotions
Work
Ambitions
Housework
Post

To achieve goals you need to set yourself priorities. There is so much choice available today that you could feel that you have somehow failed if you don't try to do it all now. However, you need to remember that most of your 'must-dos' are things that you alone have *decided* to do – they are not things that must be done. You decide to have children, a career, certain relationships, a nice house or a car because you feel they will benefit your life. Everything involves time and effort to achieve, so decide what really is important to you and what you really need to do well. You have choices to make and you need to choose if you do it now, delay it, delegate it or just dump it.

Summary

- Face Reality To Achieve Your Dreams: You can only change what already exists so use that as your starting point.
- Open Your Mind To Opportunity: Don't dwell on what you cannot change; focus on what you can change.
- Knowledge Is Power: The more you know, the clearer the solution will become.
- Make Progress In Small Ways: Look for small, manageable steps to improvement rather than hoping for immediate transformation.
- Accept Or Change: Accepting your current situation will help you make changes to improve it.

Assess Success

It is often your attitude to success that convinces you that you have achieved little. Success is a very subjective thing – what others see as successful you may perceive in a different way. Your attitude to past experiences dictates whether you categorize those experiences as an achievement or a failure. If your expectations are too unrealistic and over-optimistic then your chances of success are very slim. If you take a more realistic view, one that takes into account the limitations, lack of information and timescale available when you made a decision to act, and equate that with the result, you are likely to be much more forgiving about what constitutes success. It is hard to reach a perfect result because all our surrounding influences would need to be in perfect alignment.

To be consistently successful, you should view success not as the attainment of the perfect result but in terms of your ability to cope with a situation under the relevant circumstances. Anything that improves your situation, no matter how small, or anything that has given you greater knowledge to improve on the future, should be categorized as a success – even if the experience was an unpleasant or unsatisfactory one.

You would never deliberately choose to do anything that could have devastating results so the fact that you deem something unsuccessful after the event must be down to either your implementation of the action or your expectation of the result.

Plan To Succeed

Pretend you have already decided to act on your desire; talk yourself through it and imagine how it would work. If you envisage lots of potential pitfalls and disappointments then you are making the wrong choice or you need more information and time to prepare. It's much better to work this out in fantasy land, rather than proceed and experience disaster in reality.

Think about any successful person in history or anyone you admire today. Imagine what they had to go through to get where they are – how long it took, what they experienced and what they had to do to maintain their success.

The Route To Success

It is unlikely that the people you admire simply decided to do something successful and then found it just happened. It probably took years of setbacks and disappointments before they reached their goal and, if they hadn't been successful, they would still be frustrated and disappointed about their situation – just as you probably are now. Take any of the great inventors for example – they didn't invent the light bulb, telephone or electricity in an afternoon. It took years of frustrating research and constant cynicism from those around them. What kept them going was the fact that they could see that they were making progress. Every time they tried something and it didn't work, it offered clues as to what would work and whether it was really achievable. They were increasing their chances of success by reducing the odds of failure – by systematically ruling out what didn't work they would eventually be left with what would. Of course, they didn't always achieve what they set out to but often it led to an equally exciting discovery.

Part of the pleasure of success is the effort needed to achieve it. An achievement that involves no effort or risk produces very little satisfaction, therefore these elements have to be accepted as part of the package. However, you need to find ways of reducing unnecessary effort, risk and potential damage before you will find the confidence to proceed. Past disappointment can make it hard to keep trying. You need to know how to do it, whether you can do it and what could happen if you attempt it before you feel safe enough to make that first step.

Fear Of Failure

You were not born with a fear of failure; it is something that you acquire as you progress through life. There is nothing wrong with being afraid, in fact it is a vital safety mechanism. The problem stems from the fact that we all have different perceptions of what is and isn't dangerous. Too little fear will make you prone to accidents and too much will reduce your ability to succeed. This is why you need to keep in touch with reality, remove irrelevant associations and continually add to the knowledge in your inbuilt database.

An Example

All young children want to do what they see older children and adults doing. However, they can't just get up and walk, they have to learn to walk and this involves a lot of frustrating and fearful moments. They may fall over repeatedly but they don't think, 'That's it I'm not trying to walk anymore'. To them deciding not to walk is not an option, they simply need a little bit of extra help. Once they realize this they will attempt to stand up next to a piece of furniture or hold their arms out for support because they have realized that the chances are they will fall down again. They discover that furniture and people are useful for helping them pull themselves upright or protect them from injury – it may not be walking but it is a good step towards it and it is these incremental successes that provide the motivation to continue.

Realistic Expectations

Even an immature brain has the capacity to assess risk and accept it as part of the learning process. However, it also realizes that it can reduce the potential for harm and still obtain satisfaction from progress, no matter how small the steps. In fact it finds it much easier to do this at an early age because the process hasn't been complicated by emotional uncertainties and the insecurities of living. As far as a child is concerned, there is no other way but to keep trying.

Another important element in gaining success is feeling confident that you possess the ability to achieve the aim, no matter how much you still have to learn. You must be careful, however, that your expectations and aspirations don't outstrip what is realistically possible. For example, people with a handicap often appear to cope remarkably well with what life throws at them. This is because they embrace all their capabilities and use them to the maximum, rather than dwelling on what they cannot do.

Success can sometimes just fall into your lap but the chances of that happening are miniscule. If you want success, you have to be prepared to work for it and take risks, but you also need to understand that the route to success can often bring troubles of its own. Even if you did succeed with one of your ambitions, it doesn't mean that the rest of your life would be perfect. It is very common for successful people to inherit a whole new set of problems arising from their success, such as jealousy and envy. If your attitude to achieving and maintaining success is too black and white then your life will be a constant round of disappointment and bewilderment.

Cultivating The Right Attitude To Success

One particularly interesting method of psychological testing assesses a person's attitude to particular situations and then determines their likelihood of suffering from depression. The predictions are pretty accurate, even down to the calculating the number of years before the onset of clinical depression.

Those most likely to suffer from depression are those who

generalize and personalize any disappointments or failures. Such people will say things like, 'I failed the test because I'm stupid and all my teachers think I'm stupid.' This attitude implies that they are useless at everything, disliked by everyone and there is nothing they can do about it because that is how they are.

Those who are most likely to live a happy life are those who compartmentalize and depersonalize their reasons for failure. For example, they will say something along the lines of, 'I failed this particular test because I did not revise enough and I had a terrible cold.' This attitude assesses the reasons for failure and views it as a one-off, something that might have had a more positive outcome had they taken greater control over the situation or if circumstances at the time had been different.

We all have the ability to control our attitudes and most people can move from one category to another depending on their circumstances. If you have experienced a series of disappointments you will be more inclined to swing towards the depressive attitude – but that doesn't mean you need to stay there.

Look at your attitude – do you label yourself using negative terms that imply you cannot change things?

Do you think that is how other people see you?

Do you think they are to blame?

Do you think you have no control over your life?

Look at the people around you, what do you say about them?

If your answers indicate that you see other people as having all the power and yourself as powerless – or blameless – then you need to reassert control. You have the power to change things. If you can compartmentalize and depersonalize, then you have a much better chance of having a happy life. Just because something didn't work out once, it doesn't mean it will never work – there is still the potential to achieve success from it.

Mind Motivation

Anything with an element of risk has the potential to generate new problems. Most people find it hard to change because they know they will be upsetting the apple cart. Your cart may well be full of rotten apples but at least you're familiar with its content. Do you usually wait until your condition becomes unbearable and then force yourself to change, not really caring what you're throwing yourself into? If so, you fear change and will only take that step when the motivation to do so increases dramatically. You know you need to change but are afraid to do so because it involves taking risks, could upset people and could expose you to humiliation and criticism. Are you deliberately sabotaging your own efforts and do you strongly defend your current situation, even if you hate being in it?

If you have longstanding, unresolved problems you need to look at whether it is your body saying no or you.

Mind Makeover

Ask yourself what you are trying to achieve.

When I ask clients, 'What do you want to achieve?' they may say that they want more money, better relationships or a slimmer figure but to me that is too vague. What you need to do is strip back further and ask yourself, 'Why do I want these things, why is it so important?'

Your answer will probably be along the lines of wanting a good lifestyle, more love and affection, more respect, more energy or greater self-esteem. Now strip this back even further by asking yourself again 'Why do I want these things?' You will find that you will eventually end up with the answer 'to experience happiness and satisfaction'.

Find Your Incentive

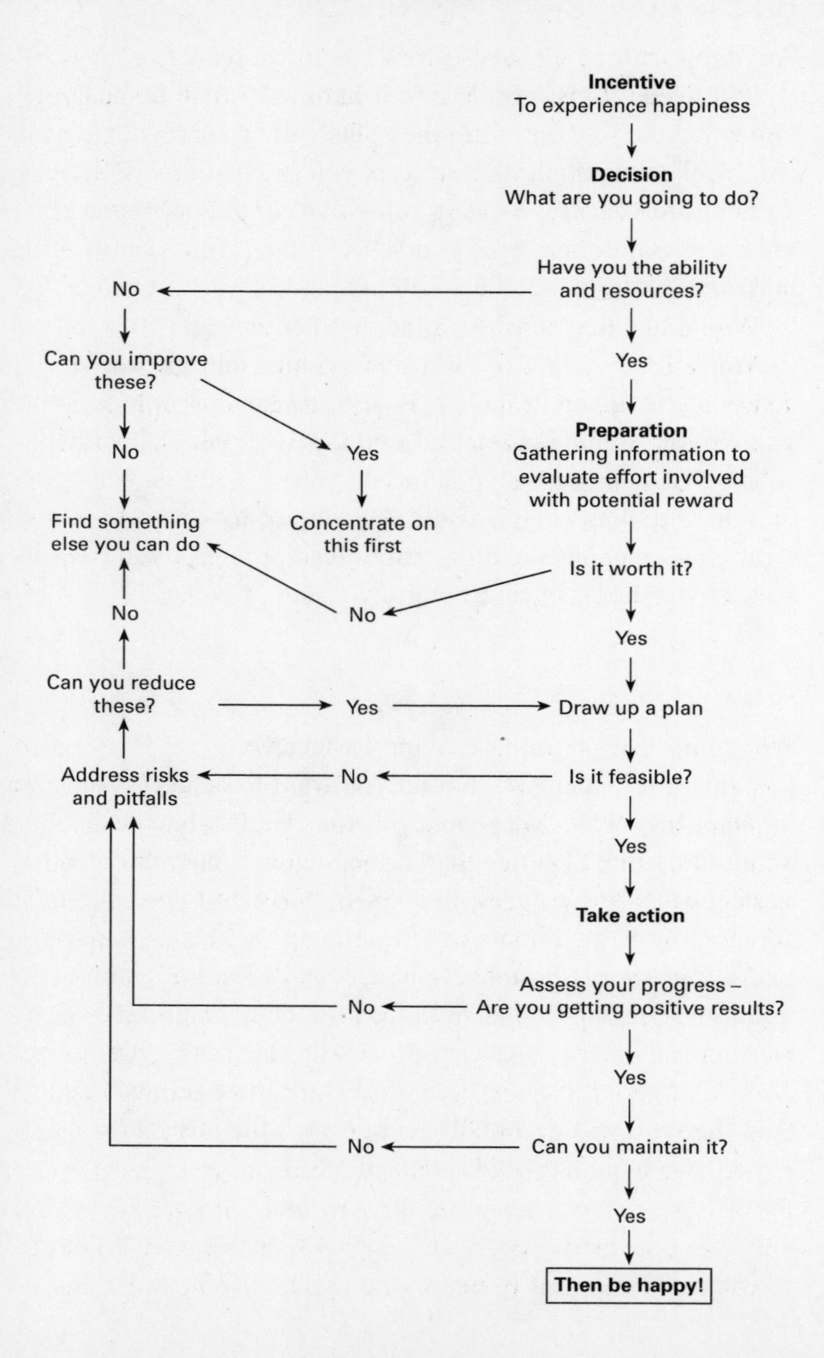

An Example

Why do you need money?

You need it to buy materialistic goods that will make living more pleasurable. You could survive in the woods by eating nuts and berries, but for most of us that is nowhere near as enjoyable as having a comfortable home with all the latest gadgets. So your motivation is to be as comfortable as possible because that makes you happier.

Why do you need to get on with other people?

You need to have good relations with people because it makes life easier to deal with, it gets things done, it provides you with respect and pleasure and all this makes you happier.

Why do you need to achieve?

You need to feel that you have achieved things and made the right choices because it gives you a sense of purpose, pleasure and satisfaction.

Recognize Your True Incentive

When you realize that happiness and satisfaction are your true incentives, it gives you a lot more scope for change. There are numerous routes to happiness, therefore you are no longer stuck with one desire. Experiencing pleasure and satisfaction is not a frivolous or self-indulgent thing, it is a biological requirement for successful living. Life is a big experiment in what will make you happy but in the process you are bound to discover things that make you unhappy – that is part of the process. These negative elements cannot be avoided and should be viewed as a reality check and a learning tool to enable you to progress. Human beings have come a long way using this process of discovering what will and won't make us happy. However, you need to accept that what made you happy in the past will not necessarily make you happy in the future – otherwise you would have no desire to continuously want to improve on your current situation.

Healthier Ways To Happiness

Research has shown that ...

- The health benefits of 20 seconds of intense laughter is comparable to three minutes of hard rowing.
- Regular brisk walking can be more effective at treating depression than chemical anti-depressants.
- You are 16 times more likely to develop panic disorders if you smoke.
- You are two and a half times more likely to have a road accident if you are obese.
- Aromatherapy can be better at reducing aggressive behaviour than traditional sedatives.

Letting Go Of Loss

When we give something up we often feel a sense of loss. This is because that something has become an emotional or physical prop. For example, giving up smoking, getting over a relationship break-up or going on a diet would be easy if the things you had to forego hadn't given you pleasure initially. The fact is they have become more of a habit than a pleasure, which is why they are now causing you problems.

To deal with loss ...

1. Accept the loss – accept that your source of pleasure or satisfaction has gone.
2. Deal with the emotions of that loss – *expect* to feel upset and angry.
3. Adjust to your new situation – adapt your life to cope without it.
4. Concentrate on making positive changes – look forward to changing your future.

Don't Be Defeated

Many of you may be feeling bogged down in a situation because you don't want to lose face or you feel that you will be seen to have lost. Frankly, neither of these things matter – all that matters is whether you are living a good life or not. We moved house once and walked straight into a typical dispute with our new neighbour over a boundary. We just sold up and moved, end of problem. Everyone said we should have fought on, shouldn't have given in so easily, stood our ground and so on. These comments probably hurt more than the disagreement because it suggested that I was a failure. To us the house wasn't worth fighting for. We bought that house purely because we thought it would improve our life but we couldn't be sure that it would. As it turned out, the move had produced a problem that we could not have foreseen and hence it had made life less enjoyable – to us, this meant the point of having the house was gone. We took a calculated risk and it didn't pay off. At the end of the day it was a box to live in and we couldn't make it into a home because we didn't feel happy or secure in it. We did the best thing for us and moved to somewhere we really did enjoy living in and could call home. To me that is a very good result because my aim was not to get into a pointless battle but to find a place I would be happy in. Eventually I found one – I just had to go round the houses a bit first.

So remember ...

- Your eventual happiness is more important than trying to win minor battles.
- It is better to work with people on an equal level than to try and overpower them.
- Offer support rather than taking control of someone else's problem.
- Tolerate those that are unimportant; don't fight for the sake of it.

Will You, Won't You?

It's all very well having an incentive but you won't get very far if you don't know how to use it. Indecision is your next point of potential anxiety because the body hates not being able to act. It is natural to feel anxious when you cannot act because you have no options. However, it can also be hard to proceed when you have too many options, because the more choices available the greater the risk of making the wrong decision. If things go wrong you could be hurt or humiliated and if that happens too many times, you will stop trying to achieve. What we sometimes fail to recognize is that in order to make progress you often need more than one option – you don't have to pick out one and throw the rest away. All your options must have the potential to get you to your goal, so if one doesn't appear to be getting you anywhere you can always try another.

If You Have Problems With Decision Making ...

1. List your options.
2. If you have more than three options, pick out the most favourable three.
3. Spend a week gathering more information on all of them.
4. Pick your favourite one and give yourself another week to focus on it further but don't do anything life-changing.
5. Assess if it is still your favourite. There are three results available to you – no, maybe and yes.
6. If the answer is yes, spend another week working out how you are going to implement it; if the answer is maybe, spend a week looking at whether you can improve it. If you answer no, dump it and go back to your list.
7. Once you have made a decision, focus your full attention on implementing that option but keep assessing and keep adding to your list.
8. After three months look back and see how your life has changed.

Things can only be classed as having failed if you have run out of options. Your 'failures' are more likely to be setbacks – although they have occurred as a result of you acting on a decision, this does not mean you have failed. You can say that particular aspects have failed but overall failure is a rare thing indeed. There is always something to be learnt from any experience in life, although wouldn't it be a better idea to be aware of the potential lesson beforehand?

Assessing The Risk

The main reason that people fail to act to improve a negative situation they are in is because they fear the risk that is inherent in change. However, life will never be risk-free and to experience life you need to take risks – there is no getting away from it. Fear usually stems from the fact that most of us have first-hand experience of the damaging effects of taking risk and we have no desire to put ourselves through it again. If this is how you feel, you need to look at how you can reduce the risk to a level that will enable you to move on. You may not be able to remove the risk but you can certainly do something to limit the possible damage to a more acceptable level.

Many of my clients are very successful in work and already know all about the principles of risk assessment. However, they fail to see that the successful systems they operate at work are no different to the ones they should be using in their everyday life. Good business systems work because they mirror the method the body uses to solve problems. Look at a work-based task: it has a deadline, it requires preparation, an objective, research, information, direction and input from external forces, and to complete it you have to have an incentive, make a decision, act on it, assess it and then get a result. These methods are designed solely to get the job done and they can be used just as successfully in other areas of our lives.

Okay so all this preparation may seem a bit tedious but if you carry out a risk assessment of any situation beforehand, it can enable you to be a lot more adventurous, because you have reduced the potential harm to an acceptable amount. Human beings love to scare themselves because it generates huge amounts of pleasure stimuli. We love roller coasters and the reason why they can be so big and so scary is because the safety aspect has been addressed. We can enjoy being scared by them without worrying about the potential harm. You don't need to experience harm to know it would be unpleasant and therefore risk assessment should be an essential part of your plan to change.

An Example

If your job involves using a ladder then you know before you go up it that it could slip or that you could fall off it. You also know that if this happened you could be killed by a blow to the head. If you fail to take any measures to protect yourself, the job will be a scary one and there will be little incentive to do it. However, if you fit stabilizers to the ladder and wear a hard hat this will reduce the risk to an acceptable level and allow you to feel more comfortable and confident in your job. This may be a simple example but it illustrates the fact that the task stays the same; it is simply made more acceptable to the person who has to do it. The preparation can be done without any change being necessary. It is only then that you need to decide if you want to proceed. At this stage the chances are you will, because your route will appear much safer and a successful result will be clearly visible. This will give you the motivation and confidence to proceed. It doesn't really matter how dangerous the situation is, it is more a question of your ability to deal with the dangers. Being prepared makes the difference between being too afraid to attempt anything and having the confidence to begin the process of change. (Have a look at the chart on page 150 as a reminder of how to address risk.)

If you are not creating a safe environment in which to proceed it's no surprise that you can't get your body to budge. It needs to know that all the safety angles have been covered and that the potential reward is greater than the potential harm. If you are stuck in a rut, risk-assess your life (see page 150) to see if this can give you the confidence you need to move on.

The Confidence Factor

To have genuine confidence you need to feel safe. Confidence can be a dangerous tool if it is not based on sound judgement, as behaving over-confidently increases the likelihood of accidents and mistakes because it denies that there are potential problems to address. There is a big difference between behaving over-confidently and being confident in your abilities. One could make things worse, while the other can only improve your situation.

You are behaving over-confidently if ...
You do not want to know what could go wrong.
You feel afraid.
You will be glad when it is over.
You hope that everything will turn out alright.

You are being confident if ...
You are prepared.
You feel excited.
You can't wait to get stuck in.
You have a plan.

A large number of the people I see feel that their biggest problem is having no confidence. Often they will say that other people see them as bright and assertive but they feel a fraud because when they are on their own they feel insecure and afraid. However, I think it is important to say that none of us are naturally confident 100 per cent of the time – we all have insecurities and fears. I get really annoyed with personality testing when it dictates that we categorize ourselves as extrovert or introvert, confident or not confident. We are a combination of all types – what you feel depends on which aspect of your life they are referring to and how skilled you are at dealing with it.

Confidence is really a tool that we all use because it could potentially produce a better outcome. If you want to meet new people or get on in life, displaying confidence will increase your chances of making a good impression. You know that if you go to a party or a job interview, you will be more successful if you promote yourself in a positive way. If you walked into a room and stated to a group of complete strangers that you had a miserable life and were rubbish at everything, they would hardly be queuing up for a chat. Even if that was how you felt, it would be better for you at this stage that they didn't know that. It would also be better for them because, underneath it all, they're very likely to be insecure too and would prefer to have confident people around them.

Be Who You Want To Be

When you first meet someone, the chances are your behaviour will not reflect your true feelings. You will present a facade and pretend to be the sort of people you think they would like you to be. After all, it is in your interests initially to do that. By appearing bright and confident, you should get a good response from them and this will make you feel good. It also means that you can find out more about them and decide if you want to form a closer relationship or just leave it at the current level. If they are behaving in a bright and confident way, the chances are they are doing the same thing. If your relationship deepens, you will feel more secure about revealing your true character – which includes your weaknesses – because you feel they will understand. A successful relationship is built upon knowing and accepting the full range of characteristics in a person and not the veneer that you first encountered.

I am sure you have met someone you initially found very interesting who turned out to be disappointingly dull the next time you got together, or you may have fallen madly in love with someone in a week and woke up a month later wondering what you ever saw in them. This sort of thing is often a result of becoming enamoured with the person they initially portrayed themselves to be, rather than the person they really are – and the more you got to know them the less appealing they became. Sometimes you start to believe the pretence and struggle to maintain a relationship based on your first perceptions, hoping that this shallow image will become part of reality. As a relationship develops and you feel more comfortable with that person, their real personality will start to show. It is at this stage that you could feel disillusionment and disappointment because, when reality sets in, things are not as glamorous as those heady early days of the relationship.

There is a theory that you should show everyone your true insecure or negative feelings. However, I believe it really only pays to be yourself with your close friends and relations. I'm not saying you should be deceitful, you just need to accept that the majority of people don't really want to know your real weaknesses because they are bogged down with their own problems and insecurities. Your nearest and dearest will take the brunt of your moans, groans and frustrations to some extent, because you know they are more likely to accept it, but imagine what life would be like if you did that to everyone. Would you really want to burden your neighbour with exactly why you are in such a bad temper or why your job is driving you up the wall – for that matter, would you want them to do that to you. No – when you bump into each other in the morning you'll smile, say hello and get into a bit of trivial chit-chat because it is important not to alienate the people around you. So behaving in a positive, confident way makes you feel better and keeps your problems on a more rational level.

Life is all about experimentation and discovery. You can never be sure of who the 'real you' is because you are always is the process of creation. This is why it pays to be positive – it allows you to continue discovering and progressing. Your aim is to turn dreams into realities – and that includes your own personality. You can be whoever you want to be and behave however you want to behave (within the boundaries of the law, of course). The simple aim then is to learn what works best for you. It is a lot more satisfying living the life of a positive, caring person, and confidence is a useful tool to help you make that happen.

Reinvent Yourself

- Smile – it will make you feel better.
- Be pleasant – it is the only way to get positive feedback.
- Focus on those you love – don't assume that they know you care.
- Watch your body language – good posture can make you look great even if you don't feel it.
- Take time to listen – you might learn something.

Remember, everyone is shy and insecure at heart – try this little exercise to boost your confidence. Every time you go to a public place like a supermarket or town centre make an effort to speak to one new person – nothing lengthy or in-depth just go and ask them the time, some directions or what time the shops close. Not too difficult is it?

If you use confidence and you get a good result you are more inclined to use it again; if you get a bad result you will be less willing to behave in a confident way because it let you down previously. So how can you make confidence work for you?

Everyone has the ability to be confident but to be successful you have to feel confident about using that confidence. To have a good chance of success, you need to reduce the fear factor and this can only come from researching your subject matter, understanding your situation and assessing the risks. If you do not fully understand what you are doing then no amount of confidence is going to stop you from experiencing a disappointing result. True confidence comes from knowing what you are doing now and what you are going to do next. A positive attitude is the result of feeling confident that your capabilities match the task in hand; it does not stem from over-optimistically hoping that things will turn out right if you just ignore current circumstances and risks.

The Pygmalion Principle

This term is used to illustrate how people react to what they believe they see and how we are capable of becoming that 'fantasy' figure, if we so choose. The principle relates to the play *Pygmalion* (though most of us will be more familiar with the musical version *My Fair Lady*), which centres around a common flower girl who is transformed into someone who could pass for a duchess. It illustrates how the way you behave and look can have a direct influence on how your life turns out; it also shows how if you work hard, keep learning, have clear but realistic goals and learn from those who have something to teach you, you can be whoever you want to be.

When you meet someone for the first time you cannot know who they are, therefore you have to make assumptions based on what you see and hear. The opinion you formulate will dictate how you behave towards that person. If you are impressed, reassured, flattered or attracted to them you will treat them in a completely different way to someone you feel is negative, weak, insecure or unattractive. However, it is incredibly easy to make big assumptions on first appearances and therefore big mistakes so it pays to tread warily.

Make The Most Of Those You Meet

1 Treat everyone with the same respect, interest and caution until you get to know them better. Imagine how you would feel the next day if you discovered that the person you met last night really did only say all that stuff about lasting love to get your pants off, or the stupid idiot you pushed out of the way yesterday happens to be the person interviewing you for a job today. An old business colleague of mine once said, 'Never be rude to someone you don't know because they might turn out to be your next potential customer.'

2 Don't dwell on your preferred perception, keep in touch with the reality.

The most quoted reason for someone staying in an abusive relationship, for example, is because 'They really love me and can be so nice when they want to be.' Of course they can, because they know that it will keep you in a situation you wouldn't normally tolerate. Real love does not involve harm or violence so there is a contradiction going on here. You cannot change something that does not exist, you can only change what is really there. This is why it is so important to understand the reality of a situation, no matter how painful. Remember that you are also being judged and assumptions are being made about you.

A negative attitude or poor body image will be an immediate disadvantage to anyone (unless they are trying to get a bed in a hospital). You may not feel great but small positive steps that encourage good feedback will make you feel much better.

3 Find yourself a role model.

Don't resent those who appear more positive, confident or successful than you, instead learn from them. Follow the example of people you admire. Find out how they achieved and overcame things – if they can do it then I'm sure you can too.

4 Surround yourself with positive people.
People with negative attitudes encourage others to develop a negative attitude because it is a form of bonding. Sometimes it can be hard to stay positive when you know those around you are waiting to say, 'I told you so.' A positive and confident attitude does not guarantee success but at least it gives you the chance of a positive result. A negative attitude gives you no chance.

Boost Your Self-esteem

Let's look at what it is that brings people together as a group. If you look at your close friends, I am sure they will all have very different personalities, careers and lifestyles. The thing that binds you together is a similar level of self-esteem. If you look at a group of people with above average self-esteem, the conversation will be predominately positive. They will discuss good times, successes and how they learnt from bad experiences. For example, there could be talk of holidays, promotion and how a recent bereavement brought them closer to their family. They will usually only discuss other people when they are concerned, proud or inspired. If someone in that group finds their self-esteem faltering due to problems in their life, such as redundancy, weight gain or a relationship break up, their attitude could start to become more negative. They will then start to become resentful of the group's successes and more inclined to make derogatory remarks about successes and failures of other members of the group.

In a group situation such as work, it often takes just one negative person to bring the self-esteem of the whole group down, with the result that other members develop negative tendencies as well. If you look at groups that stick together because they have low self-esteem, they will feel persecuted and resentful, even when this is completely unjustified. It's fine if you're happy in your little group, moaning and groaning about the world – and I have to say I have met many who are, not that they would ever admit it of course. The problem comes when you have had enough of this miserable life and you start to do something positive to change it.

Anyone in your group who does not want you to change – either because they don't want to lose your friendship or just because they are envious of you – will try to sabotage your efforts. These negative attitudes can be an important influence, one that can make it very hard for you to change things for the better.

Change Those Around You

If you were to go on a diet or give up smoking, for example, is there someone in your group who would tell you that 'one more piece of cake won't hurt', or blow smoke into your face when they know you are desperate for a cigarette?

This person will be your saboteur and they could make it hard for you to make positive changes – after all, none of us want to upset or alienate anyone at a time when we need all the help and support we can get. Do you feel that you will be forced into making a choice between keeping friends and family happy or losing them in order to change your life and make it happier?

Draw up a list of those people you *want* to have in your life, those that you have to keep in your life because of duty and those you can distance yourself from. Reassure those you are closest to and ask them for help and guidance so that you can make the change together. Accept any resistance from those you are duty bound to – they may well not want you to change because you suit their needs as you are. Distance yourself gently from those who bring you down – you do not need them in your life. New, more positive friends can be made and negative attitudes can be changed if you stay committed and positive.

Don't Get Stuck In A Victim Syndrome

It's all a matter of attitude. There is one group of people I know I cannot help and that is because they have what I call an invalid attitude. They complain about their lifestyle but choose to do nothing about it. It has to be assumed that this is their preferred option because they have no interest in changing. They know they can get attention and sympathy by complaining. If someone tells me they know everything about stress, that they have struggled all their life or they recite a catalogue of traumas and, after all that, finish with the sentence, 'But I coped with it well', I know I'm on to a loser. They don't want my help, they just want someone to tell them how fantastic they are at coping and how well they look under the circumstances. They are stuck in a victim syndrome.

I have never been a great fan of struggling. Yes, we all have to go through times of adversity but it should certainly not be something we aspire to. If someone proudly tells me their life has been one long struggle, I feel immense pity because no matter how difficult life is the thing that should make you feel proud is the fact you have managed, in spite of adversity, to achieve an element of success and enjoyment. It is very unlikely that anyone reading this book will be a professional moaner. Such people never consider reading a self-help book because – as they are only too keen to point out – they know it all. There are two good reasons why you might be finding it hard to change. The first is because you don't know how to change and the second is because you choose not too. You may have made your unhappy situation your preferred option because you see no other option that is more favourable to you. It is very rare that people are forced to stay in a situation they dislike and

usually they know what they need to do to get out of it. Nobody is forced to smoke and get lung cancer, or over-eat and become obese, therefore you need to ask yourself why,
if you are so unhappy in this situation, are you still in it?

Case History

I was once asked to advise on a seriously obese lady who was so overweight that she couldn't leave the house. I was asked what would be the first thing I would do to help and I said, 'Find out who is feeding her because if she can't get out of the house to buy food then someone must be bringing in all this food for her to eat.'

It emerged that she had become the psychological controller of the household and was getting her family to buy her all the food she wanted, even though they were the ones who should really have been in control of her diet. As unhappy as she was, she was maintaining her situation through emotional blackmail. She feared that if she lost the weight, she would be able to look after herself, thus allowing her family to go off and live their own lives. She felt they cared so little for her that the only way she could get their attention was as a dependent. She made them feel guilty for depriving her and upset them as a way of maintaining the level of care and attention. This had resulted in a destructive cycle that maintained her unhappy situation and that of her family, making her comfort-eat even more. She had chosen to be a victim and although this is often a justifiable feeling it can be counterproductive in the long run and a big obstacle to change.

It can be difficult to achieve our hopes and desires without the support of others. Getting that support can be a problem because we are all working to different rules and have our own objectives. Making assumptions is one of the biggest causes of stress and anxiety. The only thing we can assume about other people is that, deep down, they are probably just as insecure as we are. It is therefore in your interests to reassure and motivate those around you so that they will feel secure enough to do the same for you. If you say yes, then you don't want everyone else to say no.

Visualization Exercise

Imagine a corridor with 20 doors in it. There are four people who all have the same goal or dream and this just happens to be behind one of the doors. The only thing they don't know is which one.

There is a small chance that they could open the right door immediately but it is more likely that they will have to pick a few wrong ones first. This is the reality of the situation and it is this that dictates the odds of success. Technically they all have the same chance of success but there is a lot they can do to influence the outcome. What do you think the odds are of success? The odds on them opening the right door on the first go are 20 to 1 but there is no limit as to how many goes they can have, so in fact there is a 100 per cent chance that they can get to their goal if they are prepared to open a few wrong doors first. What they need to remember is that, no matter how unpleasant the consequences of opening the wrong door, it will improve their odds of opening the right door because the amount of doors left to open will have been reduced. So in reality a wrong door is not a setback, it is a step forward.

The first person goes into the corridor and happens to pick out the right door straight away – a perfect result. This is where the element of luck can feature, because there will always be a chance of getting the best result, no matter how slim the odds are. Luck is a random element that is not dictated by justice or effort. No matter how much you love luck and envy those that appear to be lucky you must remember it is a rare thing indeed and not something that can be relied on. Instead you need to improve your chances of a good result rather than leaving it to luck. Back to the corridor – the person who has picked the correct door straight away is overjoyed and goes off to celebrate, leaving the other three behind. The next person walks into the corridor and picks out a different door. Behind this door is a man who asks him a question that he needs to get right before he can move on. This person has no idea what the answer is but he realizes that he should do because it relates to his goal. This makes him feel stupid, inadequate and too fed up to carry on. He goes off, persecuting himself for being so stupid, annoyed at the previous person for having all the luck and promises himself he will never put himself through this sort of humiliation again.

Just by chance the third person picks the same door and he doesn't know the answer either. However, this person sees himself as a fighter; he is determined to get to his goal so he goes off to learn enough to enable him to answer the question so that he can go on to open another door.

The fourth person also picks this door but he knows the answer. He is no brighter than the other two but when this opportunity was presented to him he decided to do all he could to achieve his goal. He has already researched his goal so he knows all about it – whether it is worth all the effort and how he can make it easier to achieve. He has spent his time up until now gathering information and running through a few coping strategies, so it's not surprising that he can easily answer the question and move on.

In the meantime, the third person has gone off to find the second one and persuade him to give it one last go. He is very reluctant but they all give him encouragement and so he agrees to try one last door. As soon as he opens the door, he is sprayed with water and completely soaked through. For him, that is it, he now classes himself as a failure. He is humiliated and disappointed and has the attitude that nothing is worth trying again. From now on he will be miserable with the way his life has turned out and he will encourage everyone he meets to underachieve too.

Back in the corridor, the third person has, by chance, gone for the same door and he too gets covered in water. Not one to give up, he goes home to dry off and prepare himself to soldier on. The fourth person also looks at this door but he knows a lot about his goal. He knows it is warm, hot and sunny and this door is cold to touch, has mould on the framework and a puddle of water at the base. He uses his knowledge to discount this door. This means that not only has he avoided an unpleasant event but also increased his odds of opening the right door sooner.

Both he and the third person will open the right door eventually but at what cost? To the third person it has been one trauma after another but to the fourth person it has been a calculated route of discovery. He can decide if it is worth continuing because he understands completely what he is trying to achieve. The third person may tire and give up despondently in the same way as the second one did or he can carry on and reach his goal to discover it was not worth all the effort. For the fourth person, that little bit of preparation and thought beforehand meant that he could have an easier route and a worthwhile objective. If he gives up, it will be because he chose to having decided it was not worth the effort – not because he thought he was stupid or was physically exhausted from every setback.

Can you associate with any of these characters?

Have you had experiences that relate to all of them?

Have you experienced similar emotions?

Whatever your approach, it is not cast into your character; it is up to you which example you choose to follow. You will not always be lucky, but you can learn new techniques and you can improve your chances of success. The second person could regain confidence through learning, but so too could the third. The lucky person at the beginning isn't off the hook either. He could become overconfident as a result of his lucky break and suffer repeated disappointments because he thought everything would always be that easy to achieve – therefore he too needs to prepare in future.

If you want to improve a situation you have to look at your approach to it. Luck is a bonus but you cannot rely on it. We all have similar situations to face as we go through life but success only comes to those that have the right attitude towards it. Be objective and ask yourself which person fits your own approach. Look at your past successes and look at how you achieved them. Ask yourself, 'Do I want to say yes?' because if you don't then your body will always reply with a resounding no.

Try This

This is a great method of getting positive feedback.

Start a conversation with a positive statement or a compliment and see what a difference it makes.

For example, 'You are a beautiful person and that dress does not do you justice', is a lot better than 'Yes your bum does look big in it'. If someone has made a mistake, your immediate reaction may be to ask why they messed up. This naturally makes them defensive and they will blame someone or something else, feel stupid, get upset and regret ever offering to help you in the first place. However, if you start with a compliment or a positive statement such as, 'You're usually so good at these sorts of jobs so I was surprised it went wrong, is there anything I could have done to help or can you advise me on what we need to do to stop this happening again?' you remove the need for conflict, reassure them that you don't think they are a complete idiot and make them more willing to put things right and do a better job next time.

We all need reassuring and highlighting the good points makes everyone feel better about working together. When things go wrong we tend to behave as if everything is wrong.

Reaffirming the existing good elements and isolating the problem reduces the likelihood of conflict in irrelevant areas and focuses on resolving the actual problem. A positive approach enables you to deal with conflicting views without creating emotional insecurity. It always helps, when stating a difference of opinion, if you make it clear that this does not affect the love, care or respect that exists in the relationship. In fact, it can strengthen it by demonstrating a desire to work together as a team to resolve future problems and differences.

State The Complaint

Not everyone is easy to get on with, even if you shower them with compliments. If you find it hard to deal with people because they are negative or aggressive, for example, it could be because you are responding to them in a way they recognize and expect. Although you may be having different conversations about different topics, the pattern of response could stay the same. For example, if someone is always complaining, your reaction may be to agree because you are not that interested and it keeps the peace. You may be fed up with their continual moaning but it is your response that is encouraging them to continue.

Try This

If you are fed up with a continuous negative response then state your complaint. For example, if someone is negative about everyone and everything then, rather than mumbling in agreement, respond by saying, 'Are you all right? Because it is not like you to be so negative' or 'I remember when you used to be so positive, it was great then'. Of course it is 'like them' to be so negative but a lot of their negativity is due to the fact that they have developed a pattern of conversation they think is appropriate when they talk to you. By responding in a different, more positive way, you will have broken the expected pattern of response with the reassurance that you will continue to speak to them, if they change the pattern. This gives them an opportunity to assess their own attitude without the insecurity of criticism and gives you a chance to vent your frustration without causing conflict.

You may feel that you are being deceitful by pretending to be nice to someone you don't like or by telling someone they are not unpleasant when they are, but once you give it a go you'll find that they are much easier to be with and not so bad after all. Anyway, if you get a good response from being positive, it will soon become part of your nature to behave that way and not a façade.

Make It Easy

Life is difficult enough so your aim must be to make things as easy as possible. That is what evolution is all about. We now have washing machines to do our laundry and we don't have to rely on the nearest stream, and thankfully we have supermarkets to supply our food so we don't need to hunt big scary animals. There are no medals for anyone who wants to live their life difficult so if you have a problem to solve, take the route of least resistance.

If you follow the logic of the brain and prepare, assess and implement a safety plan then you will find an easier path to recovery. If you use all the techniques and equipment your body has available to build confidence, ability and positive attitudes then you will find the help you need to succeed.

Let's look again at how the body likes to operate. It needs to feel that the effort required is going to be worthwhile. It likes to take the easiest, not necessarily the shortest, route to success and it needs knowledge and ability to give it the security to succeed. Once you have all that then your body will want you to say yes.

Summary

INVEST IN EFFORT – accept that it could take time to achieve success.
MAKE A DECISION TO ACT – don't add to your anxiety by dwelling on what could go wrong.
ASSESS THE RISKS – address them now to reduce them in the future.
USE CONFIDENCE – it will bring you more positive feedback.
TAKE A POSITIVE APPROACH – reassess your attitude to success.

Part Three

plan for success

It can take a long time to become unhealthy or unhappy, so the chances are it will take time to recover. We all have different reasons why our health and happiness is affected and this is why you must experiment to find out what suits you personally. This is what I mean by experimenting with change. If you suffer from chronic or repeated health conditions you need to question whether you are doing anything to maintain them: is it your lifestyle, your attitude, your diet or that pint of strong black coffee you have every morning?

You need to look at everything, no matter how small or trivial it may seem, and assess if it is having a negative effect on your body. It may well be that the 'can't live without' props you insist on having every day – the things you think keep you going – are adding to, or even maintaining, your continuing problems. For example, I see quite a few people who insist they cannot give up smoking because they will put on even more weight – but they are already overweight and smoking so to me it doesn't seem like a very effective form of weight management. In fact, their smoking is probably indirectly adding to their weight gain because it is dramatically reducing their energy level and draining the body of nutrients, creating a constant craving for high-calorie foods.

So what practical steps can you take to improve your own well-being and bring your body back to a healthy balance?

Recovery Plan

Now it's time to take a close look at your five-point combination plan.

1) How can you run your stress response right?

The golden rule to follow in order to avoid harming your health and well-being is not to do anything to extreme, for too long. In part one we looked at how the body needs to be run to stay healthy and in good working order. It likes to be stimulated through motivation, it likes to make quick decisions, act immediately, get a result, assess and then rest. The reason why this is so important is that there really is no other way of running it effectively and successfully, therefore, if you want to be able to cope with the stresses and strains of living and feel good, you have to abide by the rules.

Tips to improve motivation: Try the '48-hour' exercise in part two and recognize your true priorities and incentives. You need to discover what is really important in your life before you will find the motivation to change.

Tips to improve decision-making: Try risk assessing your life to remove the fear of change and accept that making mistakes is a part of making progress.

Tips to increase activity: Try the 4D exercise in part two to get you organized and focus on the benefits of your actions.

Now look at an average day in your life – are you running your body according to the rules?

Write down everything you did in one day. How did you feel by the end of the day?

If you felt happy and satisfied then you are running your stress response well. If you felt exhausted and miserable you need to look at how, by making small adjustments to your decisions, actions and incentives, you can use your stress response to improve the outcome of your day.

2) How can you encourage positive stimulation?

Pleasure and satisfaction are essential requirements so it is important that you experience them. You need to make time to have fun, to be with those you love, and to achieve, otherwise your life will be full of regret and unhappiness. Be aware, however, that you may not be recognizing the existing satisfaction you have in your life because of your approach and attitude to the situation you are in. In part two we looked at how you can change your approach and attitude to situations to bring about a more positive result, why it is important to get on with people and make a positive impression – go back and re-read this section if you need to refresh your mind.

The best pleasure and satisfaction is experienced when you are in the best possible health so the advice in part one on keeping your body healthy is vital if you want to keep those wonderful, natural happy drugs flowing. Maintaining good health should not be dull and boring but having poor health and being unhappy certainly is.

Things to help you feel more positive:

Look for the benefit in everything you do.

Learn from your disappointments.

Behave in a positive and confident way, even if you don't feel it.

Put your energy into what is really important.

Make time to have fun and to do nothing.

3) How can you incorporate relaxation?

If you want to lead a stimulating life, you need plenty of genuine relaxation. Balancing stimulation with relaxation is vital and breathing techniques and short relaxation breaks can help to keep the responses healthy (see part one). You also need to consider changing those aspects of your life that could be having a detrimental effect on your energy levels and physical health.

Great ways to relax:

Have a massage – Either book a weekly massage or do self-massage. Using an oil, gently stroke your arms, legs, shoulders, neck and temples. The key is to stroke towards the heart as this helps to clear toxins and excess fluid from the system.

Do some deep breathing – Deep breathing is the basis of good relaxation and you can do it anywhere so make sure you incorporate it into your day.

Try positive visualization – It isn't easy to empty a troubled mind so instead think of something pleasurable or positive, such as a favourite place or person, any positive thought will give your body a breathing space.

Sleep properly – A good night's sleep is essential as this is the time your body does all its major work. Prepare your body for bed by writing down anything that is worrying you or has to be done and tell yourself you will look at it again in the morning. Don't eat or drink anything stimulating for about two hours before you plan to go to bed and try to go to bed and get up at the same time every day. Generally, the best quality sleep happens before midnight so watching television until late into the night is not going to be very beneficial.

Lack of sleep and relaxation can have a devastating effect on your health as it means your body cannot keep up with essential maintenance and repair. A US study found that if they deprived healthy young men of four hours sleep a night for only six nights in a row, their blood test results matched those of a diabetic. So as you can see, it pays not to mess with your body's natural cycle.

Engage in low-level activity – Reading a book, going for a walk or taking up a sport such as tai chi, Pilates or yoga all encourage relaxation. Each, in its own way, takes you out of your everyday concerns and allows you time to switch off.

4) How can you put the right resources in?

In part one we looked specifically at how diet affects health but what is important now is discovering how this is relevant to you. In order to do this you need to list how you have, up until now, dealt with your own health and well-being issues and start to assess this. What makes you feel good, what makes you feel worse, is there a regular pattern? – these are the sorts of questions you need to ask.

It is not just a case of putting the right resources in but of making sure that your body is capable of processing them. This is why it is so important that you take a combined approach if you want optimum health.

The key to a healthy diet is...

Balance
Variety
Pure foods
Foods that release energy slowly
Low intake of stimulating foods
A good mix of fats, carbohydrate and protein
Foods high in minerals and vitamins
Plenty of water
Avoiding anything that upsets your system

5) How can you keep harmful substances out?

It is impossible to keep out all harmful substances because we absorb and breathe things in all the time. However, a healthy body is equipped to deal with a certain amount of such abuse. What it finds difficult to handle is the onslaught of excessive amounts of toxic and over-stimulating substances, combined with on-going stress and anxiety. It appears that many of us are on a route to self-destruction, deliberately subjecting our bodies to things we know damage our health or even kill us prematurely. As I have demonstrated throughout this book, this is not necessarily because we are weak-willed, it has more to do our natural healthy balance being so consistently upset that it has forced the body to resort to desperate measures to keep it going. There's no question about it – if you want to get the balance back these harmful substances have to go.

Ways to beat the cravings ...

Join a self-help group.

Find some healthy ways to have fun.

Take up a hobby.

Make a positive change in another aspect in your life.

Set yourself a goal.

Prepare an effective plan to overcome them.

Spend more time in the fresh air.

Find some healthier friends.

Focus on how much better you will feel.

Starting Point

The stress chart in part one is designed to determine what sort of stress you are suffering from and which direction you need to take to find your line of contentment. If you are still not sure which type of stress you are suffering from, the following lists will provide further clarification.

Passive Stress

Most likely if you ...

Find it hard to motivate yourself

Feel better when you achieve something

Feel better out of doors

Suffer from anxiety

Worry all the time

Feel tired all the time

Are overweight

Stimulants and eating make you feel tired
Are bored or fed-up
Suffer from low self-esteem
Feel disinterested a lot of the time
Feel bitter about the way life is
Sleep loads but still feel tired

If you suffer from passive stress, a combination of positive stimulation and quality relaxation should be your preferred route to recovery.

Active Stress

Most likely if you ...

Always seem to have a crisis going on
Have sudden losses in energy
Feel exhausted when you are not busy
Never have time to eat properly
Always have lots of 'must dos'
Find it hard to switch off
Feel worse after exercise
Depend on stimulants and live off fast food
Feel angry and irritable
Tend to overreact
Find it difficult to get a good night's sleep

If you suffer from active stress, your body needs relaxation and physical care to help with restoration.

Identifying the type of stress that you suffer from will give you a starting point for your plan of recovery.

Putting It All Together

To make improvements, you need to ask why things have not improved.

What has stopped you so far? For example, if you are in an unhappy relationship, why are you still in it if it is making you so unhappy?

These are the sorts of questions you need to ask:

- Is the unhappiness in the relationship a symptom of an underlying cause like a sudden loss in income or problems with the children?

  You would then need to consider ...

  How you could stop these negative issues from affecting the positive elements of the relationship.

  Could you use this experience to strengthen the relationship or to give you the incentive to start a new life somewhere less stressful?

  These lines of thought will help you formulate a positive plan of action rather than feeling that you are powerless to act.
- Is the relationship the cause of your unhappiness because it has broken down or because your partner is unpleasant or selfish?

  You would then need to consider ...

  How happy does this person really make you feel?

  Are you facing the reality of the situation?

  What commitments you have that prevent you from walking away from the relationship.

  You then need to look at how you can make your immediate situation more acceptable and make it a priority to invest some of your time in making a long-term change.
- Is your problem a symptom or is it the cause?

  In part two we looked at the importance of preparation because before you can start solving a problem you need to first assess if that problem is a cause or a symptom. Let's use weight gain as an example. This is really a symptom, but a symptom of what? It could be unhappiness, a physical disorder, lack of positive stimulation, just sheer over-indulgence or a combination of all four. Unless you deal with the underlying issues then the symptom will continue to exist and cause you further problems. If you know the cause of your problem you need to look at why you have been unable to resolve it so far or, if it is incurable, how you can make it more tolerable. What is your symptom trying to tell you?

Is your body trying to tell you to change your pace of life, change your diet, change your attitude or seek medical attention? If you cannot deal with the cause, what other things can you do to help your health and well-being?

Making any positive improvement to your life will give your body a helping hand towards better health. You may have to accept that some things cannot be changed, so focus on those things you can change for the better. Remember, everything in your body and mind is interrelated so even if you think it has no relevance to your problem, any improvement you make will still have a positive effect on it.

Top Tips To Get You Started

Ask For Help

- Always consult an appropriate health professional before doing anything else.

  For example, don't assume that your lack of energy is just down to the fact that you have been working extra hours or that your loss of concentration is just because you are getting older. Always get things checked out with the people who are there to help. If they can't find anything wrong, don't be upset, it could be your body giving you a warning sign and that means there is still time for you to do something constructive about it yourself. Don't ever feel intimidated by health professionals, they are there to help you and they will be only too pleased to know that you are taking an interest in your own health as it only makes their job easier. Do, however, keep them informed of any self-help measures you're planning, as they may well be able to help you further.

- Look at all the various types of help available.

  The majority of complementary therapies work because they encourage the body to relax and heal. They are perfect for maintaining good health and for dealing with the effects of stress on the body. Unfortunately, people often only turn to them when all else has failed and then expect them to be a miracle cure. In such demanding circumstances they could appear to be ineffective, but in general they can bring a huge amount of relief to a sufferer, as well as helping to prevent health problems. Regular massage, for example, breaks up toxic waste, making it easier to dispose of, which in turn reduces the amount of stress on the body. Similarly, many people believe that the only benefit of essential oils is that their nice smell helps you to relax but did you know that oil rubbed on the skin only takes about 20 minutes to reach the liver?

  This is why it is so important to understand how your body works. If you understand its needs it will be easier for you to assess what help and advice will benefit you and what is irrelevant or even potentially harmful.

Boost Your Body Image

- Look at your posture, how good is it?

  If it is not good then you are putting unnecessary physical strain on your body and sending out negative signals that could influence the way people respond to you.

- Look at your appearance, what signals are you sending out?

  Taking care of your appearance may seem an insignificant thing when you feel awful but natural beauty care is not just the preserve of the vain. It is a preventative health measure and a way of dealing with negative symptoms at an early stage. For example, your skin likes moisturizer because it stops it from cracking up and your hair likes to be washed because it helps keep it free from harmful bacteria. The fact that these things also make you more appealing to your fellow human beings is a feel-good bonus.

A study at Yale University showed that just having a bad hair day or not washing your hair was enough to send self-esteem plummeting and self-criticism soaring. When you think about it, who needs thousands of pounds worth of research to tell them this? After all, what's the first thing you want to do when you've been ill in bed for a few days? Wash your hair!

- Think about your body language, how often do you smile?

  Okay so you may well not have a lot to smile about at present but your body likes to smile, it gives it a glimmer of hope and encourages those feel-good responses you so desperately need. It also gives you a greater chance of experiencing a positive reaction from other people – and that is bound to cheer you up.

Get Informed

- Gather as much information as possible in the time you have available.

  The more you know about your subject, the more confident you will be about tackling it. By staying informed, you can continually assess your situation by asking yourself if you are going in the right direction, if it is working, if there is something better available now that you understand it more, if it is still what you want, and if your goal is still attainable.

  The more you know, the more confident you will be to experiment and the more capable you will be of dealing with things when they don't always turn out successfully or go to plan.

Be Active

- Make activity part of your everyday life.

  Activity should not just be an add-on to enable you to stay fit for living an inactive or unhealthy life. Your body prefers to keep moving all day rather than have the odd sudden burst of activity – and it likes to have a reason for doing it.

  Gyms were not around when the human body was first put together; it was designed to be used in the process of living so ask yourself how much do you actually move? Think of increasing your activity level by walking further, buying a bike, doing something while you are waiting for the kettle to boil or photocopier to print, taking the stairs and walking the kids to school. Look at how much people move when they are enjoying themselves, talking passionately and taking part in something they love doing. Exercise will give you a buzz and keep you fit – but only if you enjoy it and have the time to enjoy it. If you hate going to the gym or have to go there at 10 p.m. because that is the only time you can fit it in, then you are only stressing your body out even more.

  Increase your level of daily activity, such as taking the stairs instead of the lift and so on, and buy a step meter to monitor and improve your levels, or find an active hobby that you enjoy doing. For example, joining an amateur dramatics group may not initially seem an obvious way to keep fit but it has all the right qualities. You need to get there, you will be moving around all night, using lots of different muscles, you'll be doing something other than eating, be more aware of your body image and experience positive stimulation. If you enjoy that and loathe the gym, then for you it's going to be a better way to get fit because you will want to do it regularly, make time for it, look forward to it and get positive stimulation from it.

- Look at everything you do as a way of increasing your fitness as this will encourage you to be more active in the way you go about your daily life.

Create The Right Environment

- Look at your environment to see what could be detrimental to you and if you can either improve on it or remove it.

  Look at the people around you; are they supportive towards you? People that judge and criticize you are probably just as insecure as you think you are and you are on a loser if you attempt to keep up with their high expectations. Don't even bother trying, instead concentrate your efforts on creating a more positive atmosphere. You don't need to and can't be friends with everyone but don't go out of your way to alienate. Only negative results can come from being negative. If you behave in a positive and pleasant way there is a chance that you could benefit from the outcome.
- Make your lifestyle manageable by de-cluttering all your life – your possessions, the people around you, your 'to-do' list. Don't get bogged down with your past but keep it precious by preserving it in a containable memory box – and make sure it only contains happy memories.

  Any change, no matter how good, will always involve an element of loss. This is often the reason we find it hard to make a change. You may grieve for chocolate if you go on a diet and cigarettes if you give up smoking. Accept that a small loss is often necessary to bring about a positive change. Remind yourself that you don't have to give anything up or change anything forever, you can always go back – but would you really want too?
- Set your own benchmark for success because people will always exaggerate how popular they are, how successful they are and so on, and the fantasy rarely matches the reality.

And anyway, what use is someone else's idea of success? Find your own route to happiness rather than trying to keep up with the competition.

Get A Grip On Reality

- Remember, you can only change a situation if you have grasped the reality of it.

  Results and solutions can be perfect but the majority of the time the reality will involve a measure of compromise. Look for an improvement rather than having unrealistic expectations. The best results come from taking steps to improve on what is real. Improve on reality now and you have a chance to make perfect dreams come true in the future.
- You have a choice to either accept your situation or change it.

  No one is making you pile on the weight or is preventing you from taking time out, for example, it is you – you are doing it to yourself so find out why you are stopping yourself from improving your life. The reality is that everyone has chores and responsibilities but that doesn't mean that you can't change your approach and attitude towards them and make them more manageable and acceptable.

  What is the best that can happen if you don't make changes to your life?

  Ask yourself what happens if I don't do it?

A Balanced Plan

So you have now decided what you need and want to change and you are ready to make that change. Now is the time to make it happen.

To put together a plan of action you first need to look at your priorities – what do you need to change first? I find it helps to start off with a short-term plan with a time scale of three to six months. This will address those immediate issues that centre around the state of your health and well-being. Once you have got to grips with this, you won't need to devote so much time to it and you can move on to a life plan to help you build a better future.

The reason I like to concentrate on health first is because if you are feeling tired, run down, fed up or bogged down with chronic health conditions, you are not in the best state to do anything. Concentrating your energies into health restoration will renew your energy levels and improve your emotional and physical states, all of which will make a big difference to your ability to succeed. You may find that many of your problems are due to the state of your health and will therefore disappear when it improves. You will also find that any remaining issues will be easier to address because your renewed energy and ability to see things more clearly will enable you to deal with them effectively.

Step One

Take four pieces of paper and write one of the following headings at the top of each one.

Chores and Duties
Health and Well-being
Pleasure and Passion
Goals and Ambitions

Under chores and duties list all the chores and duties you have in your life. Under health and well-being list all the things you think you could do to improve your health and well-being. Under pleasure and passion list all the things you think you would really enjoy doing. Under goals and ambitions list all your dreams and desires for the future.

Dealing With Chores And Duties

A balanced life contains aspects from all the above headings, so if your life is imbalanced you are probably overloading on chores and duties and neglecting all the others. You will probably find that some things on your list overlap. For example, if you have children, unless you have perfect little angels, they should, I would have thought, fit into both chores and duties and pleasure and passion. There is no getting away from the effort involved in bringing up children but the more they feature in the pleasure and passion zone, the happier you and your children will be. Chores and duties have to be an accepted part of having children but the reason why you wanted them is because you thought they would benefit your life and of course they should be doing just that.

There is effort involved in everything you do but the positive results it produces should mean that these things are not a burden to you. Unfortunately, because chores and duties are often unavoidable and reoccurring, they tend to dominate and the pleasure and passion element is often neglected. Your priority now is to make as much time as possible available to make life good. This means that you need to take steps to make your chores and duties bearable and contained so that you can focus more on the pleasure they should bring.

Most people find that 80 per cent of their life is a combination of chores, duties and mundane living, therefore it is vital that you make the most of that precious 20 per cent. A great way to deal with your chores and duties is to use the 4D exercise in part two (see page 151), because many of those chores don't all need to be done that well, or even at all, they just need to be sorted as quickly and efficiently as possible so that you can go out and enjoy life. As an example, let's look at a particular chore that not many of us claim to enjoy – the ironing. Normally what happens is that you avoid the ironing until the airing cupboard door refuses to close. You may have been avoiding it for days, even weeks, before you're finally forced to tackle it. By this time you already have that little nagging voice in your head chanting, 'must do the ironing, must do the ironing'.

This little voice makes you feel inadequate because you can't get your head round a simple task like ironing, so what chance have you of getting anything more complicated sorted out. To add to that, it is a constant source of stress because you are not dealing with it. Finally, you have had enough of this irritating little voice and decide to do the ironing when you get home that evening. But of course you can't be bothered so you go through another couple of days of it burning a hole in your mind until you finally give in. This sort of niggling irritation may only cause low-level anxiety but if you combine it with all the other 'must-do-but-not-got-round-to-yet' anxieties and thoughts such as 'must go to the gym, see my mother, change my boring job ...' it all adds up to a continuous amount of serious stress that is a real strain on the body. Not only that, these on-going anxieties dominate your thought processes so you never have a clear head to think about important changes and improvements in your life.

To start to bring this mayhem under control, before you do any task you should ask yourself why you need to do it. You need to actively *choose* to do chore or duty before you can get the motivation to carry it out. So, for example, you are choosing to do the ironing because you prefer to wear smartly pressed clothes in order to create a better impression and feel good about yourself. No one is forcing you to do the ironing, you prefer to do it because it is gives you the opportunity to get a better result. You therefore cannot ignore the fact that if you want your clothes to look good you need to do the tedious task of ironing, simple as that. There is nothing you can do about that fact but you can do a great deal to either reduce it or make it more tolerable – and, more importantly, reduce the anxiety this unimportant task causes.

You could, for example, reduce the amount of ironing by buying clothes that don't need ironing, you could pay for someone to do it, get the person who's ironing it is to do some of it, or you could reduce the unpleasantness of the task by arranging to watch your favourite television programme at the same time.

Another approach to finding a solution is to look at things from a different angle. If you put 'not doing the ironing' on your ambitions list it could motivate you to get a better paid job so you can pay someone else to do it or encourage your partner to help out more. Having to do the ironing should never impinge on you achieving pleasure and satisfaction in your life. If you want to have a better life then anything that plays a part in preventing that has to be addressed.

Time Allocation

Once you have attacked your chores and duties list in this way, you should have a clear picture of what really needs to be done – and if something has to be done then you need to make time for it.

Now is the time to put a plan together – you can either do this in your diary or divide a sheet of plain paper into seven sections to make a week. You won't always have to be this methodical because once you know what you want to do and what needs to be done, you will just make it happen. However, when you are trying to incorporate new things into your life and want to see the progress you have made, it pays to plot it in black and white.

Allocating time to a chore or a duty will prevent it overflowing into you life and removes that constant anxiety of knowing it needs to be done. To demonstrate, let's continue with the ironing example and imagine you have reduced it as much as possible and don't dread doing it so much. Now you need to allocate an amount of time to enable you to keep on top of it. First assess how much ironing you accumulate every week and if, for example, it takes an hour, find an hourly slot in your week that most suits your schedule and arrange to do it then.

sample plan

Monday	Tuesday	Wednesday	Thursday	Friday	Saturday	Sunday
Work Practise micro breaks	Work	Work Keep practising micro breaks	Work	Work	*1 hour* Sort out finances. How much can I save for holiday? *Study hour* What job would I like to do? Look on internet to get some ideas Make shopping list and menus Arrange to start diet on Fri Clear out wardrobe	Keep clear to enjoy *Shortlist:* *Good weather* Drive to sea Have barbeque Lie in sun and read *Bad weather* Lie on sofa and read Have a pamper day Go to pictures
	Lunchtime – check out shops for healthier things to eat		Lunchtime – phone friend	Take 20-min walk in park		
	Walk home from work	Pop in to see Mum on way home				
90 mins housework	20 mins relaxation break when you get home	Ironing hour 7–8	Try out new dance class	TV night – do nothing		

Priorities

Short term — improve diet; more relaxation; have day out with friends

Long term — round world trip; find more job satisfaction

Set everything up at that time, work on it for exactly one hour and then put it away. If you have a backlog, then build in a bit more time until it is clear but think about the necessity of ironing each piece as you pick it up. If it has been un-ironed for any length of time you obviously don't like it or need it.

By putting your chores and duties into a schedule, you are removing the anxiety of not dealing with them therefore that little voice will stop nagging you. If you put this hour into your schedule, you can also see how much time is now available to you, so by containing your chores and duties you can free up time to do the things that will ultimately make you happy. If you do this with all your chores and duties, obviously your week will start to fill up but even if you are only left with an hour free at the end of the week, it is still an hour you may not have thought you had. An hour to relax, an hour to make plans, an hour to learn or an hour to have fun, rather than an hour spent thinking there's something you should be doing but you can't quite think what it is.

I am always being told – usually by some disorganized person who is bogged down with endless chores – that planning takes the fun and spontaneity out of life. In fact, it increases the likelihood of it because it allows you to put pleasure and satisfaction first. If they are your priority, then you are making time for them around the necessary but tedious parts of living. Planning in time to have fun, achieve or just do nothing seems much more appealing than hoping that these things will appear while you are avoiding some tedious chore. It also gives you something to look forward to. Having a schedule means you can change it at any time because it was your choice to arrange it like that in the first place. If someone phoned you just before your ironing hour was about to begin and said they had some free tickets for a great show, you're not going to turn them down because you need to do the ironing. Having a structure to follow means that you can go out and enjoy yourself knowing you can reschedule your chore and not feel guilty about not doing it that evening.

I know that the ironing is a very simplistic example but the method of resolution is the same for anything that needs to be sorted in your life, even complex problems. I am not just talking about physical chores and duties, it applies just as well to emotional issues. For example, look at the people in your life, if there are some who fit more in the 'chores and duties' category than the 'pleasure and passion' one, can you see how you can use this coping process with them?

Often it is the people around you – work colleagues, family and so-called friends – that are an emotional drain on you. Do a '4D' assessment of them and if you can't just dump them find out how you can limit the damage they cause. Make it your choice to continue seeing them by fixing regular but limited times to have contact. Make sure you arrange this in advance so that they fit into your schedule, rather than you being dominated by theirs. Making an arrangement also stops any anxiety and guilt brought on by avoiding them and this makes you feel less resentful. It also stops them nagging you because you are showing them that you care. Once you have arranged to see them, think of something pleasurable to do with them. If you find their company difficult, refuse to respond to their negativity and arrange beforehand to do something that is pro-active, like going to the cinema or helping with the decorating. Finally, keep your expectations realistic because if they have never been pleasant or very supportive then this is what you should continue to expect. Don't live in hope that they will suddenly transform into the person you always wished they were.

Step 2

Now that you have dealt with the tedium of life and made it manageable, you need to start making plans for a better life. Let's start with your health and well-being. Whether you want more energy, to be slimmer, fitter or happier you are going to have to dedicate some time to making a difference.

Improving Your Health And Well-being

There are so many things to choose from so where do you start?

First you need to write a list of all the things you think you could do that could potentially improve your health and well-being. You then need to relate this to your specific limitations and your environment – so there's no point, for example, deciding to take up surfing as a way to keep fit if you are landlocked in the middle of the country because it won't be feasibly possible to do it regularly enough. If you have a passion for surfing then moving to the sea could be one of your ambitions but it is not going to get you fit in six months. Equally, there is no point forcing yourself to go jogging if you hate doing it or your body is not up to it.

The point of having a list is to illustrate how many options you have available so that you can never say there is nothing you can do to change your situation. You are not supposed to try everything on it all at once, its purpose is to show you all things you can do. You need to pick out one or two favourites and concentrate your efforts on doing them well. Go back to your five-point combination plan. You need to find something you can do to help you balance stress, something that will help you generate positive stimulation, something that will help you relax; you also need a new healthy eating plan and a plan to detox your system. So, for example, to help you relax you could set aside half an hour a day to do some deep breathing and visualization exercises, your healthy eating plan could be the one listed in part two that follows a set time scale, and you could organize yourself to give up smoking. You can then allocate time to comfortably fit these things into your schedule and concentrate your efforts on them rather than being awash with this, that and the other.

If you continually assess your progress and set review dates in your schedule you can plot your chosen course of action to assess if it is working. This gives you an opportunity to decide if you want to continue or if you think it would be better to go back to your list and try something else. This is your process of experimentation and it should be an evolving thing because the more you experiment, the more you will learn about your subject matter. Some things may not initially work but they may introduce you to new things that do. Don't get bogged down with something just because you promised yourself you would do it – if you find halfway through it isn't working or you don't really enjoy it as much as you thought, then give it up. Your process of discovery will help you to discover new ideas, new places and new people who are more inspiring to be with.

Initially this may seem like a lot of work but, in your short-term programme, you are concentrating all your effort on a priority and at this point in time there is nothing more important than your health and well-being. Once you have your plan of action it should be easy to implement if you plan it over time. Even if the time you spend on changes only amounts to a few hours spread over a week, or just ten minutes here and 20 minutes there, these small steps will add up over time and give you the confidence to be more ambitious as you see progress. When you find something that works, the chances are it will become a natural part of your day-to-day life so you won't need to remind yourself to do it. So, for example, you will automatically find yourself stopping regularly for a micro relaxation break because you know it's the best way to boost your energy, or you will find yourself cooking healthy food without too much effort. And once such things become second nature, you can start to invest more time in the next things to achieve, resolve or improve.

Look for things that make you feel happy and healthy and accept that you don't need to do everything now or all at once, you need to work through it in stages. There is also no need to make dramatic changes to your life, often a change in approach or attitude is enough. So it can, for example, be good to have a night vegging out in front of the telly – as long as it makes you feel relaxed and you are not doing it day in day out and feeling guilty and anxious about it. It is also perfectly fine to put your plans to sail round the world single-handed on hold because you just want to take life at a slower, more enjoyable pace. You can always resume your ambitions again in the future – but only if you want to.

Step 3

So let's finally move on to the two categories that will form the basis of your plan for life. You have allocated time to get rid of the drudgery and time to keep yourself in good health, now you need to consider what will inspire you in the future – your pleasure and passion, and your goals and ambitions. These are essential elements of long-term good health and well-being. Your short-term plan was designed to improve your overall health and well-being. Three months should be enough time for you to notice a difference and six months should see you comfortable with your new health regime. This means you can divert some of your new-found energy into the final stage of your life plan.

Again, it is all down to preparation. Although your focus in the first six months of your plan was on your health and well-being, this should not have meant you neglected these four essential elements. In your quest for health and well-being you will have been making time to enjoy positive stimulation so your pleasure and satisfaction levels should already be higher. Also, this time will have given you an opportunity to think about what is really important in your life and where, for you, true happiness lies. Preparation is essential to enable you to focus on what your pleasures, passions, goals and ambitions are, or could be, and if you don't know then now is the time to find out.

Pleasure And Passion

Make a list of all the things that have the potential to make you happy, make you laugh or make you feel good. You are looking for things to do that may have no purpose other than to generate these feelings, therefore it could be a one-off thing like a day's shopping with the girls, watching your favourite comedy film or a day at a theme park. It could be something that you need to plan for the future, like a trip to Australia or having a spa bath fitted in the garden or it could be something you do on a weekly basis like setting aside time to play with the children or getting your partner to give you a full body massage. The point is, there doesn't have to be a point, you just choose things that you look forward to doing.

If you remember the 48-hour exercise we did in part two, this is a great way of demonstrating how simple pleasures are the most memorable and achievable, and how real happiness lies in how comfortable you feel with yourself and those you have around you, so this is a great starting point for assessing what makes you happy.

There will be things on your list that need a bit of long-term planning so select one and concentrate your energies on making that happen. You can go back to your list at any time if it isn't working out. Remember, if you do your preparation, you can decide if it still looks as good once you have had time to investigate it further.

Also on this particular list will be things that you can do at a whim, depending on what you feel like. This is where you can enjoy a bit of spontaneity, because if you find you have a bit of spare time or just feel like a break you have a whole range of things available to you that will brighten your day. You do still need to plan a time to enjoy life, even if you don't know yet how you are going to fill that time. Plan into your schedule blank times so that you have time booked in which to indulge yourself – you can then choose what you fancy doing at the time. This way you can make time to spend with your friends, partner or family but have the additional excitement of doing what you want, when you feel like it.

Goals And Ambitions

These are slightly different from your pleasures and passions because they involve a lot more time and effort to achieve. In addition, the process may not always be pleasurable, although perhaps it will be more satisfying in the long run. This can be anything from building a sailing boat and sailing round the world in it, to writing a novel, living in a little cottage by the sea or making sure your kids get a good education.

It can be a long-term ambition that will involve years of time and effort, such as training for a new career, or a short-term goal such as decorating the living room. Again, you need to draw up a list and then pick just one short-term goal and one long-term ambition because you don't want to drain your energy and dilute your ability by trying to do too much at once. You will only experience success if it is really achievable so there is no point setting yourself targets that are unattainable in your current circumstances – although part of your plan could be to improve those circumstances.

You need to make time to achieve goals and ambitions without swamping your life with too many things to do. Selecting and focusing on one will enable you to do that because even spending just half and hour a week on a project can help you achieve a lot over time. Often dissatisfaction and unhappiness is generated from just not giving yourself time to think things through. If you give yourself that small amount of time every week you may find that there is enough satisfaction in your life as it is, without having to go out and conquer the world – you just never had the opportunity to sit down and recognize it. Once you find out your true priorities in life you will see how little you really need in order to be happy and life will automatically became less complicated. Then you can have a full and active life, achieving goals and ambitions and experiencing pleasure without the need to plan it all out so methodically every week. If you introduce something new into your life, a plan will act as your guide and security blanket but once it becomes part of your life, it becomes your natural way of living rather than something you must remember to take the time to do.

Remember, your lists and method of planning are there for you to come back to when you need a change, a new idea or to help you decide which direction to take next so keep it evolving by adding new ideas and removing those that are irrelevant. Planning to change will give you choice, control and the power to change. It will also mean you are less inclined to cling to things that are making you unhappy and unhealthy.

Time To Go For It

The rest of your life is ahead of you and the responsibility lies with you to make it as happy and healthy as possible. You should be living your life in the pursuit of happiness and to achieve that you need to have good health. If you want your life to change then you need your body to help you. If you want to say yes and your body is saying no then you need to listen to what it is telling you. Work with your body and it will always be happy to say yes.

resources

PIC
Spearmarsh House
Almeley
Hereford
HR3 6LQ
Tel: 070 00 783694

For details of Liz Tucker's courses and programmes.

Yorktest Laboratories
Murton Way
Osbaldwick
York
YO19 5US
Tel: 0800 0746185
Email: clientsupport@yorktest.com
Website: www.yorktest.com

For information on food intolerance testing, recommended by the British Allergy Foundation.

British Complementary Medicine Association
PO Box 5122
Bournemouth
BH8 0WG
Email: infor@bcma.co.uk
Website: www.bcma.co.uk

For information on finding a qualified complementary practitioner.

Quit-Line 0800 002200
Website: www.quit.uk

Help and support to give up smoking.

Drinkline 0800 9178282

Advice and information on alcohol consumption.

Liz Tucker has a private clinic to enable her to give individual help and she also runs a whole range of health days and courses throughout the year. Her one-to-one programmes *Lifespace* and *Weight Matters* are held every month at Champneys Health Farm in Tring.

Lifespace

Lifespace is of particular value for those suffering from stress-related illnesses, typically involving chronic fatigue, low self esteem and confidence, anxiety and control issues, lack of motivation and happiness, chronic health conditions and the signs of 'burn out'. Many of you will have felt unwell or unhappy for some time, trapped in a downward spiral of physical ill-health or emotional unhappiness that makes you fearful for your future health and well being.

Lifespace aims to break this seemingly inevitable decline through a greater understanding of how problems occur, helping you to deal with negative elements in your life so that you can focus on a happier, healthier future.

Weight Matters

Weight problems are a symptom that the healthy balance of your body has been upset. This imbalance can produce not just a weight imbalance but a whole catalogue of other conditions such as food cravings and compulsions, digestive disorders, bloating, fatigue, intolerances and sensitivities. These physical problems can then create feelings of unhappiness, anxiety, dissatisfaction, fear, loss of control and poor body image. All this can have a devastating effect on your overall health and well being.

This programme looks at weight-related problems, with the aim of showing you that it is possible to get to grips with your weight. Plenty of advice and a range of coping strategies are covered throughout the programme to enable you to plan a new you.

Understanding Food Intolerance

> One of the major factors in the restoration of my health was diet. It seems so obvious now, but it took me a long time to find any beneficial help and advice. Having a greater understanding enabled me to find the fast route to good health.

It is often easy to spot an allergic reaction but if the reaction is due to an intolerance, then the vague symptoms and delayed onset can make the diagnosis difficult and often an intolerance diagnosis is overlooked.

There are many reasons why our health can be affected by what we eat and drink and an intolerance is just one of them. *Understanding Food Intolerance* not only explains food intolerance theory but also looks at reasons why you could be having an adverse reaction to food.

If you are suffering from a chronic or seemingly untreatable condition or have felt generally unwell or fatigued for ages, for no good reason, then this down-to-earth book could help you decide if a food intolerance is seriously worth addressing as a possible route to recovery. *Understanding Food Intolerance* is full of help, advice and information to help you make better choices about your health.

£6.99 inc. post and package, mail order only (tel: 070 00 783694).